BREAST CANCER REVOLUTION

A reference guide to optimising your quality
of life during and after Breast Cancer

Jen McKenzie

BREAST CANCER REVOLUTION

Welcome to Breast Cancer Revolution

As part of your purchase you have been granted access to The BCR Resource Vault.

All you need to do is scan the QR code on this page and then input your email address and name and you will be redirected to the vault.

The Vault will house the videos of the exercises mentioned in the book as well as many other video, audio and written resources to help support you as you read the book. You will also find links to Jens various online platforms and your invitation to a private facebook group just for buyers of the book.

Please Scan the QR code above

Fill in your name and email on the web page and you will be good to go.

Hello and Welcome

Congratulations on taking a powerful step towards your health and well-being by purchasing the First Volume of Breast Cancer Revolution!

I'm Jen McKenzie - The Breast Cancer Physio. I hold multiple qualifications, including being a Lymphoedema Physiotherapist, an ESSA Accredited Exercise Physiologist, and a Co-Founder of The McKenzie Clinic, an Allied Health private practice situated in Queensland, Australia.

Deeply committed to improving referral pathways to Allied Health services after a breast cancer diagnosis, my expertise lies in treating breast cancer patients and providing support for resuming everyday life during and after breast cancer treatments.

Please acompany me as we delve into the complexities of Breast Cancer and work towards achieving your optimal health following surgery, chemotherapy, and radiation.

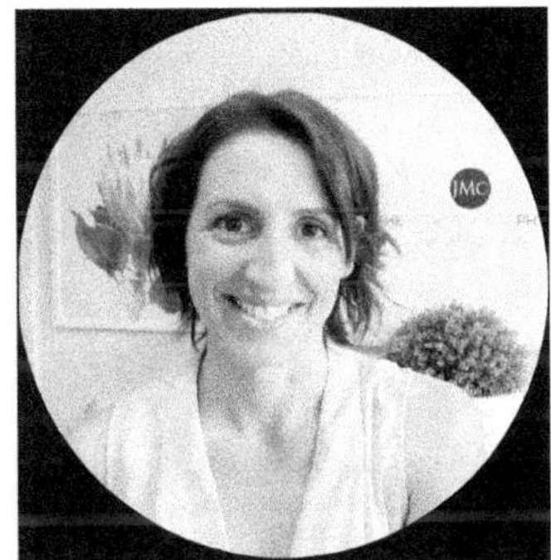

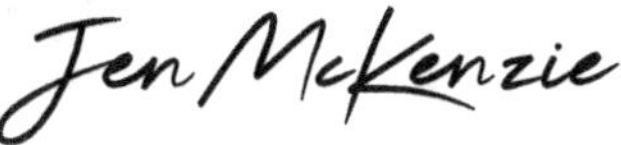

Founder, The Breast Cancer Physio

Sunshine Coast
Queensland
4556
Australia

ISBN: 978-969-44-9251-3

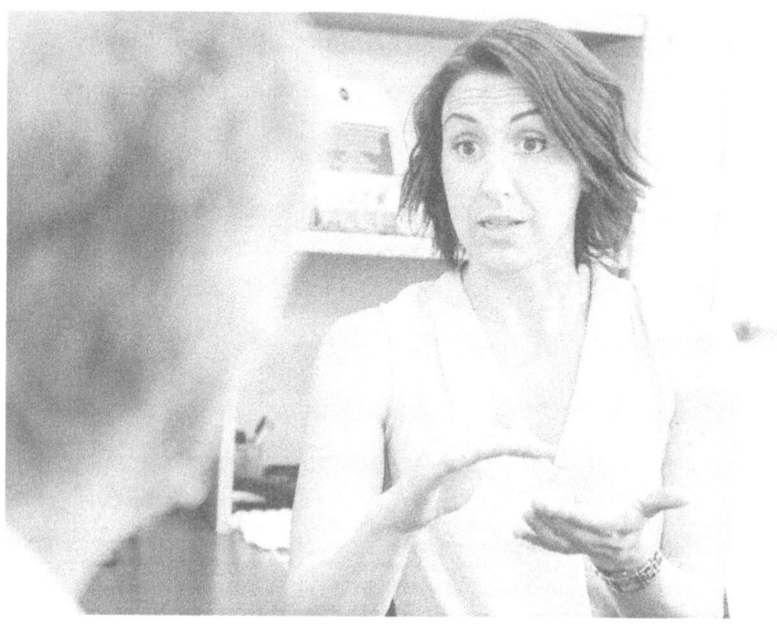

THE
BREAST
CANCER
PHYSIO

www.BreastCancerRevolution.co

"You have Breast Cancer".

So many women have expressed to me how they felt, when these words were spoken out loud for the first time. When you hear you have Breast Cancer, it's as if time has frozen. There is life as you knew it before these words, and there is life after these words.

These words change a woman's life forever. And often not just her life – the lives of family, friends, and loved ones around her. In most parts of the world, if you've been diagnosed with Breast Cancer you can access adequate to outstanding, comprehensive Medical Care. You may have already had breast surgery, you might be halfway through chemotherapy, or you may be out the other side of radiation treatment. Many of you may be planning breast reconstruction surgery or starting Hormone Blocking Medication... All these treatment options are typically available to women in many countries around the world. By the way, if you're someone who finished Breast Cancer treatment years ago and has just found this book – keep reading, it's still for you. But more about that later.

Breast Cancer is becoming increasingly prevalent around the world. Current statistics show that since the mid-2000s, women diagnosed with invasive Breast Cancer has increased approximately half a percent each year. In 2020, it was estimated that worldwide, over 2.2 million women were diagnosed with new cases of Breast Cancer (ASCO, 2023).

There are many factors and theories that may contribute to the increasing prevalence of Breast Cancer. But the overwhelmingly positive news is that survival rates, particularly for those women diagnosed with early Breast Cancer, are improving dramatically (ASCO, 2023). So, while the incidence of Breast Cancer is increasing, the risk of dying from Breast Cancer is decreasing. This is not to disregard the tragic fact that people are still dying from Breast Cancer every year.

Significant leaps in medicine are enabling women to survive Breast Cancer across the globe more than ever before. This is a phenomenal achievement by the medical community and deserves considerable recognition and accolade. To survive is to be given more time. More time with family, friends, and loved ones, and this indeed, is a precious gift.

And yet, despite this incredible outcome that women are living longer after a Breast Cancer diagnosis, we are faced with a secondary problem: due to the marked improvement in Breast Cancer survival rates, we now have a significant and increasing number of women across the globe, who are living, and struggling, after Breast Cancer treatment. Not thriving...only surviving.

If you're reading this book, chances are, you've been diagnosed with Breast Cancer, or you have a loved one that has been diagnosed with Breast Cancer, and you're desperately searching for answers.

But answers to what?

Answers to questions that extend beyond the Breast Cancer itself. Answers to questions about "all the other stuff" that is not the Breast Cancer, but essential answers that will allow you to carry on with your life, get back into activities you *must* do, and return to activities you *love* to do. Answers that will mean you can reduce pain, start moving, get stronger, return to work, look after your children or grandchildren, sleep through the night, and settle a lot of the anxious thoughts running around your head.

We're talking about *treatment side effects.*

It doesn't take long for anyone who is being treated for Breast Cancer, to become aware of the significant number of side effects – physical, mental, emotional, financial and psychosocial. Side effects that are not only significant in number, but also significant in how they impact your quality of life.

The worst part: these side effects are often not mentioned, validated, discussed, acknowledged, or addressed by a lot of Health Professionals who – you thought – were supposed to be supporting you through this incredibly traumatic time. Have they supported you? Absolutely! They have literally saved your life. But there seems to be a lot of missing information.

You are confused. If there are so many side effects of Breast Cancer treatment, why is no one talking about them?

It becomes clear over time that your Medical Team are not even able to address or treat your growing list of side effects. This is not to say you should not report your side effects to your GP or Breast Cancer Specialists. But I must point out that for the majority of treatment side effects, your Doctors are not actually performing treatment - they need to refer you to Allied Health Professionals. Medical Professionals deal directly with the cancer and its treatment. They do not deal with the *side effects* of Breast Cancer treatment.

Notably, this information should be made clear to all patients diagnosed with Breast Cancer. It would certainly sort out a lot of confusion earlier in the journey. But it is not.

A caveat to my point. The above comments do not apply to *all* Medical and Health Professionals. Many Health Professionals around the globe provide comprehensive education to their Breast Cancer patients on side effects of treatment and triage their patients onto the appropriate Health Professionals that can treat said side effects. However, in my clinical experience over the last decade, there are literally thousands of Breast Cancer patients and survivors consistently reporting the same issues from all over the world: lack of attention to, and management of, treatment side effects. I know this because I talk to these women every single day.

We have a global problem. And I would like to start to help solve these issues.

So, this is the aim of my book: *to provide comprehensive education on the side effects of Breast Cancer treatment so that you feel validated, empowered, reassured and in control. Not only provide education but inspire you to believe that - despite one of the most traumatic experiences a woman can go through in her life - with the right education and support, you too can thrive after a Breast Cancer diagnosis and continue your life in an even more fulfilling and wholehearted way following treatment.*

There are literally hundreds of thousands of women around the world, that are putting up with treatment side effects because they were never referred to the right Health Professional. And in all honesty, in previous years that Health Professional didn't even exist! It is a relatively new concept that we can have Physiotherapists, Physical Therapists, or Occupational Therapists specialising in the care of Breast Cancer patients.

Unfortunately, Allied Health Professionals and Breast Cancer are not words that have been associated with each other until more recent years. And even now Allied Health Professionals specialising in Breast Cancer care are still having to fight for their role to be recognised.

You may be reading this book years after your treatment has finished but you are *still* dealing with chronic side effects of treatment. This book is still for you. I have treated women 5,10,15 and even 20 years following their Breast Cancer treatment. Whilst I may not always completely resolve symptoms after many years, I can still provide symptom relief. We can still improve quality of life

You may have been diagnosed with Stage IV Breast Cancer. This book is still for you. Just because your disease is incurable and ongoing treatment is required, side effects of treatment can still impact your quality of life, and you still deserve to have focus on quality.

I can already feel the guilt of my readers drifting into these pages as you read this text... You are supposed to be grateful to be alive. You are not supposed to complain. About anything. You just survived Breast Cancer. What else could possibly matter? Many of you will have experienced the shame when you dared to ask your Medical Professionals about a certain side effect of your Breast Cancer treatment, only to be told that you need to 'learn to live with it'.

They may not have voiced an opinion on said side effect, but rather expressed body language that suggested how ungrateful you are to be concerning yourself or them with complaints about your new symptoms. You know exactly what 'that look' on your doctor's face means: 'I've just saved your life and you want to tell me you're unhappy?' Again I note, not all Medical Professionals have this response when patients report symptoms.

Well, I have a different way of looking at this.

If there is one thing working with women on a daily basis for the last ten years has taught me, it's this: Women are incredibly stoic and resilient, but so often to their own detriment.

Listen up ladies! Let me start this book by stating this: it is my firm belief that women do not need to tolerate persistent side effects of Breast Cancer treatment especially when – for most of the time - there is a potential solution to the problem, whether it be good management or even resolution.

I'm here to tell you a few things after a decade of experience working with Breast Cancer patients:

- You are not alone with your anger or frustration regarding the lack of attention and care for treatment side effects.
- Thousands of women around the world are experiencing the same side effects as you.
- Not nearly enough Medical or Health Professionals working with women diagnosed with Breast Cancer are providing educating on the plethora of side effects caused by treatment for Breast Cancer.
- Many of the side effects that you are suffering from are common, explainable, treatable, and manageable and sometimes completely resolvable.

And most importantly...

You can be grateful to your Medical Team for saving and extending your life after being diagnosed with Breast Cancer. And at the same time, strive to comprehensively rehabilitate your mind, body and spirit in the aftermath of Breast Cancer treatment by attending to side effects, so you can recover your quality of life, get back to doing what you love and create version 2.0 of yourself and thrive off the back of one of the most traumatic periods of your life.

Women diagnosed with Breast Cancer can, and should, be given permission to hold both outlooks at once – you can be grateful to be alive AND have high expectations and standards about your quality of life.

Providing comprehensive rehabilitation to women diagnosed with Breast Cancer has become my lifelong passion. I want this book to bring awareness, validation, education and reassurance for women all around to world who have undergone Breast Cancer treatment. I sincerely hope the words in these chapters inspire you to go after a life of purpose, quality and thriving. The Medical community have done, and continue to do, an outstanding job of extending the lives of women diagnosed with Breast Cancer. Now it is time to increase the focus on quality – not just quantity. It is time for a culture change. It is time to raise awareness and expectations.

Let's start your revolution.

BREAST CANCER REVOLUTION

Jen McKenzie

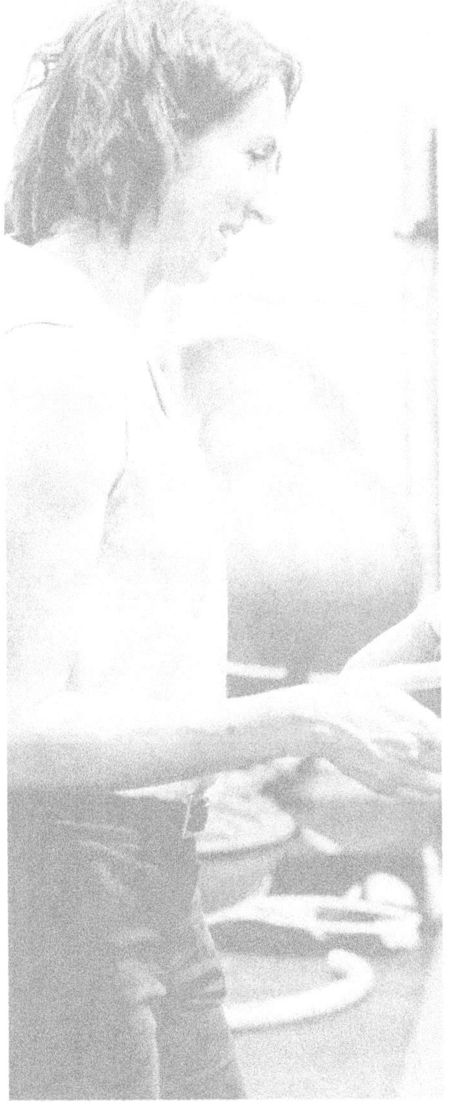

Healing Hands:

The Essential Role of Physiotherapy in Breast Cancer Recovery

1.1 Empowering Breast Cancer Recovery through Physiotherapy

Welcome to the heart of our exploration, where we delve into the pivotal role of physiotherapy in breast cancer recovery. Drawing from my daily interactions in the clinic, we will traverse through the top 10 issues that frequently emerge in the journey to conquer breast cancer. These issues shed light on the hurdles faced and exemplify how physiotherapy becomes a beacon of support, guiding patients toward recovery and renewed strength.

So many of my patients diagnosed with Breast Cancer express how they wish they had been referred to Physiotherapy earlier by their Medical Professionals or Breast Care Nurses. Earlier referral to Physiotherapy provides comprehensive education on the side effects of treatment as well as reassurance that so many of the symptoms you are experiencing are normal and common following Breast Cancer. But first and foremost, connecting with a Physiotherapist should equate to improved quality of life sooner. Physiotherapy is not typically something associated with Breast Cancer, so a referral from Medical Specialists, Breast Care Nurses and General Practitioners is vital.

01 Safeguarding Against Lymphoedema

Embarking on our journey, we spotlight the paramount concern of lymphoedema prevention. Lymphoedema, a is a potential side effect of breast cancer treatment, which can potentially occur following lymph node removal or radiation to lymph fields. This condition leads to chronic upper limb or arm swelling, chest wall swelling or breast swelling, a persistent reminder of the treatment's impact.

The risk of Lymphoedema as a side effect of Breast Cancer can be one of the most anxiety-provoking issues a Breast Cancer survivor faces. Focusing on what you can do to prevent Lymphoedema, and potentially reverse early-onset Lymphoedema, will put you in a position of empowerment, rather than constant worry and concern. Learning about how you can reduce your risk of Lymphoedema and strategies you can use to prevent Lymphoedema will assist in reducing anxiety around this impactful side effect.

Lymphoedema prevention should be a cornerstone of patient care. One pivotal strategy emerges to navigate this crucial aspect: obtaining a pre-surgery L-Dex score. (Literally meaning you obtain an L-Dex score before you have had any surgical procedures such as lymph node removal performed).

L-Dex, a shorthand for Lymphoedema Index Score, provides insight into the state of your lymphatic system. A pre-surgical L-Dex allows us to assess your lymphatic system before any surgical procedures have tampered with it. The L-Dex Score is obtained using the the Impedimed SOZO® Digital Health Platform which is a bioimpedance spectroscopy device – a bioimpedance spectroscopy device. At the time of writing this book, nowhere near enough women diagnosed with Breast Cancer are being made aware of the importance of a pre-surgical baseline L-Dex. Medical Professionals and General Practitioners could play a pivotal role in reducing the incidence of Breast Cancer related Lymphoedema if they referred newly diagnosed Breast Cancer patients for pre-surgical L-Dex scoring. I encounter many women diagnosed with Breast Cancer who, later on in their journey, wish they had been informed about a pre-surgical baseline L-Dex.

The L-Dex assessment is a pain-free test that offers a snapshot of your lymphatic system's health in 30 seconds. This baseline becomes a reference point, enabling a comparison with post-treatment conditions after lymph nodes are removed or fields are radiated.

For those ready to embrace this proactive approach, seeking the expertise of a local lymphoedema therapist with the Impedimed SOZO® Digital Health Platform". is vital. This skilled professional can perform an L-Dex Test and interpret the L-Dex score. For those unable to access a practice equipped with the SOZO® Digital Health Platform device, an alternative approach awaits. Engaging in circumferential arm measurements presents an avenue to understand your arm's dimensions before any potential onset of lymphoedema.

Research has found the Impedimed SOZO® Digital Health Platform to be superior to using a tape measure (Ridner et al 2022), however, in the absence of a SOZO device, it is still worthwhile to obtain baseline circumferential measures using a tape measure. Further to this, people with a pacemaker, defibrillator or neurostimulator are unable to use the Impedimed SOZO. For this group of people, obtaining arm circumferences with a tape measure is a valuable alternative.[1]

By connecting with a Lymphoedema therapist, be it a nurse, occupational therapist, or physiotherapist versed in lymphoedema, you can take proactive steps to obtain an L-Dex score. If you are not sure where your closest Impedimed SOZO® Digital Health Platform device is located please visit Impedimed's website www.impedimed.com and click on the Patients link and 'Find a Provider'.

These efforts illuminate a path towards lymphoedema prevention, showcasing the profound impact of informed action in fortifying against the challenges that breast cancer treatment may present. Lymphoedema can become one of the most frustrating, costly and chronic side effects of Breast Cancer treatment. Every effort, particularly early effort, towards prevention will pay dividends.

By connecting with a Lymphoedema therapist, be it a nurse, occupational therapist, or physiotherapist versed in lymphoedema, you can take proactive steps to obtain an L-Dex score.

By connecting with a Lymphoedema therapist, be it a nurse, occupational therapist, or physiotherapist versed in lymphoedema, you can take proactive steps to obtain an L-Dex score. If you are not sure where your closest Impedimed SOZO device is located please visit Impedimed's website www.impedimed.com and click on the Patients link and 'Find a Provider'.

These efforts illuminate a path towards lymphoedema prevention, showcasing the profound impact of informed action in fortifying against the challenges that breast cancer treatment may present. Lymphoedema can become one of the most frustrating, costly and chronic side effects of Breast Cancer treatment. Every effort, particularly early effort, towards prevention will pay dividends.

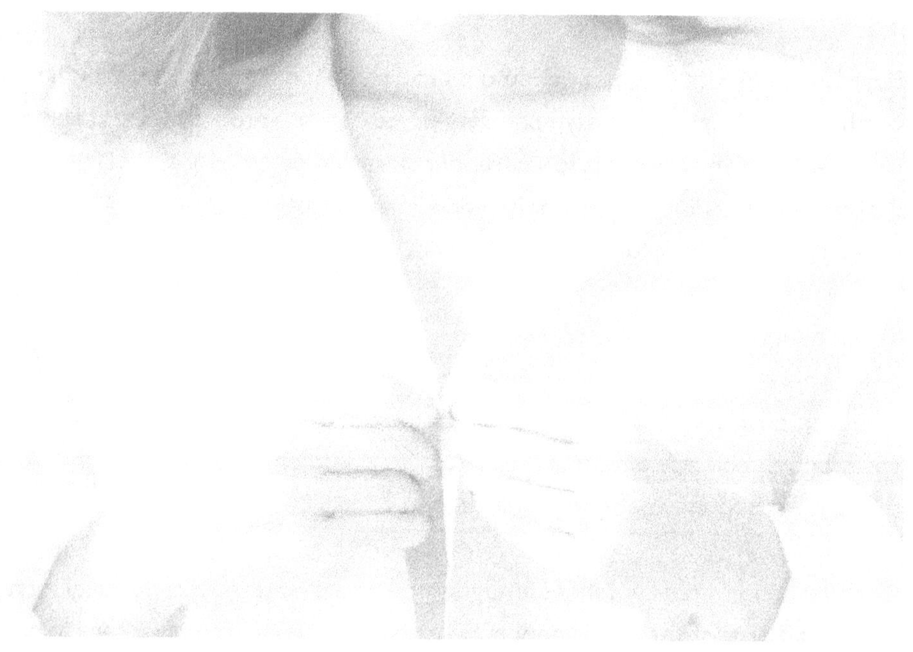

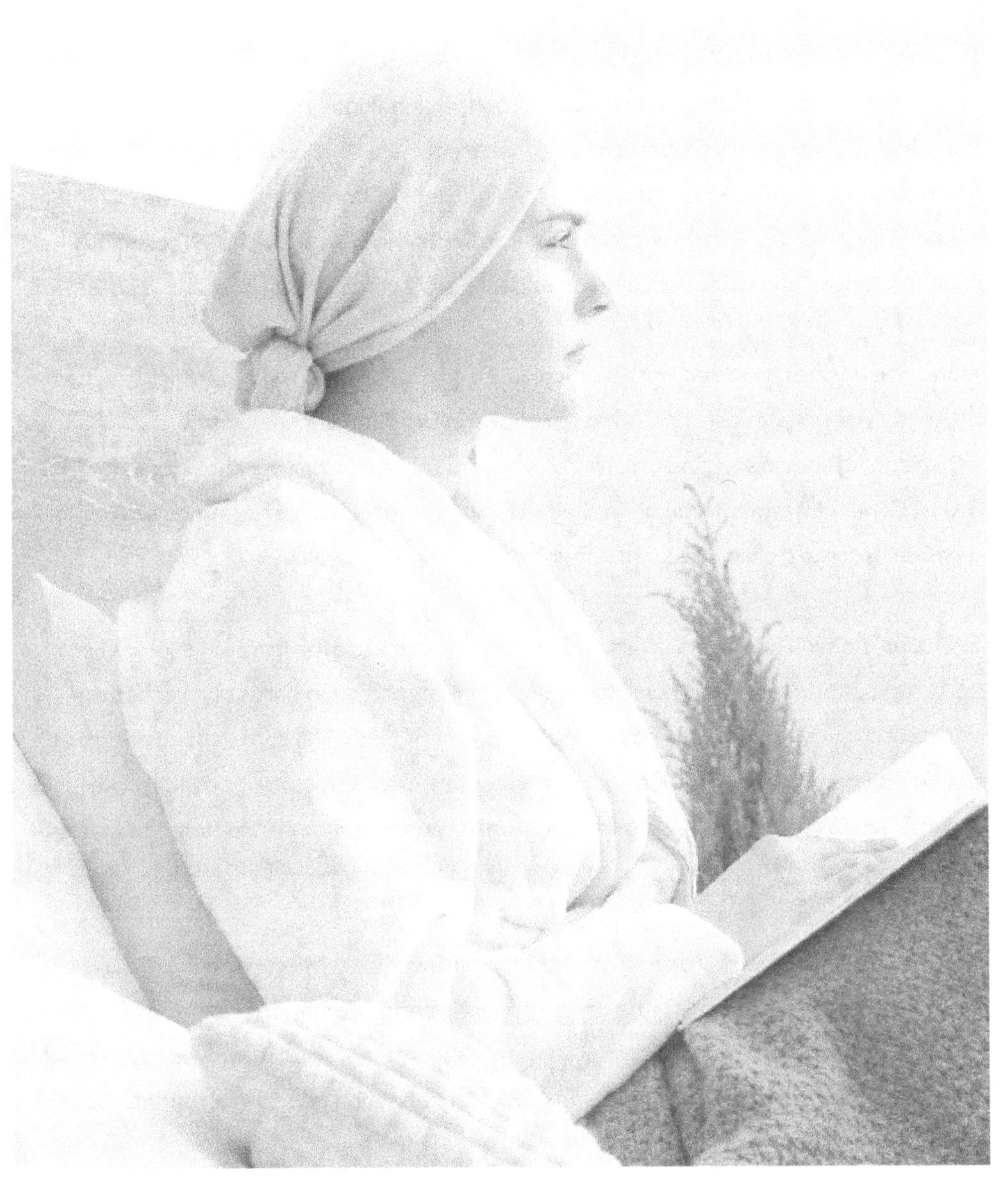

02 Restoring Shoulder Mobility

Despite the fact that most of the medical procedures for Breast Cancer involve the breast, chest wall and armpit, there is a direct and significant impact on the shoulder of the affected side (the side that has undergone treatment for Breast Cancer). The extent to which shoulder problems can occur following Breast Cancer treatment catches many patients by surprise. I often explain to my patients that the shoulder is (consciously or subconsciously) "drawn forward" in an effort to protect the breast and/or the chest wall.

Many patients are provided post-surgical mobility exercises. However, these exercises do not solve persistent shoulder issues following Breast Cancer treatment. If you are experiencing shoulder pain or restricted range of movement in your shoulder following Breast Cancer treatment, you are not alone! This is one of the most common side effects that can become a chronic issue if left untreated.

Shoulder mobility is often also limited due to side effects of treatment such as lymph node dissection scar tissue, cording, armpit swelling, radiation burns and other side effects of surgery such as seromas (trapped pockets of fluid). The combination of armpit discomfort and tension, coupled with the protective "drawn forward" position of the shoulder leads to further dysfunction and weakness of the shoulder. In turn, this can lead to issues such as shoulder bursitis or adhesive capsulitis (otherwise known as Frozen Shoulder)".

Restricted shoulder mobility becomes especially pertinent for those considering radiation therapy, which requires raising the arms above the head. Limited shoulder mobility post-surgery can lead to discomfort during these treatments and may even cause a delay in commencing Radiation treatment if the shoulder cannot be placed in an optimal position.

Restricted shoulder mobility becomes especially pertinent for those considering radiation therapy, which requires raising the arms above the head. Limited shoulder mobility post-surgery can lead to discomfort during these treatments and may even cause a delay in commencing Radiation treatment if the shoulder cannot be placed in an optimal position.

The significance goes beyond immediate discomfort. Effective shoulder movement is crucial for maintaining lymphatic flow and vital for preventing lymphoedema – a common concern after breast cancer treatment. The lymphatic system has no major "pump" of its own, meaning it relies heavily on regular muscle contraction to assist the movement of lymphatic fluid. If the shoulder is significantly restricted or shoulder pain is persisting, lymphatic flow may be compromised.

Moreover, restricted shoulder mobility affects daily life – from grooming to carrying bags, from picking up grandchildren to returning to your pre-cancer strength training program. Seeking support from experienced physiotherapists or occupational therapists is crucial. They can assess your range of motion and develop tailored strategies to restore mobility and enhance overall well-being, ensuring you can easily engage in everyday activities. Treatment for shoulder restriction is often as simple as massage and a targeted stretching program. In my clinical experience, hands-on therapy (also known as manual therapy) can make significant and rapid improvements in shoulder mobility after Breast Cancer surgery.

03 Unraveling Cording

Cording is yet another side effect of Breast Cancer surgery that is not given enough attention. Women being operated on for Breast Cancer would benefit from more education on cording even if it is only to reduce the anxiety and concern around this condition. You may be quite shocked to lift your arm following your operation and find a thick, very visible 'cord' in your armpit or even along the length of your arm. Sometimes cording can present in the breast, side of the chest wall or even into the abdomen.

At the time of writing this book, surprisingly, the medical literature has not yet defined cording. Some health professionals believe it is vascular or lymphatic structures, but from all of my clinical experience, I strongly suspect cording is nerve tissue under extreme tension.

Cording often appears as a thick cord-like structure, often presenting in the armpit. Although sometimes not visible, this condition can induce pain and impact the entire arm. Tensions may radiate beyond the armpit, leading to soreness along the inner elbow, wrist, and even the fingertips. Some patients describe tingling in their hand or fingers when the cord is under tension.

Should you encounter cording, seek guidance from a specialized physiotherapist versed in breast cancer care. They can diagnose this condition and initiate neuro mobilization exercises-a highly effective approach for cording resolution. While cording may resurface intermittently, I take solace in the fact that my experience attests to its successful resolution in countless patients. Patients are often naturally concerned when cording reoccurs, but this is common and the initial treatment techniques can be reutilised.

By becoming educated on why cording occurs and applying effective treatment strategies, you can restore comfort and mobility in the upper limb and upper body relatively quickly.

04 Addressing Scar Tissue

As we continue our journey, we concentrate on scar tissue, another common and often under-discussed side effect of breast cancer treatment. Following surgery, your body may bear various scars, including those left behind by lumpectomies, mastectomies, drain sites, portacaths and even breast reconstruction treatments.

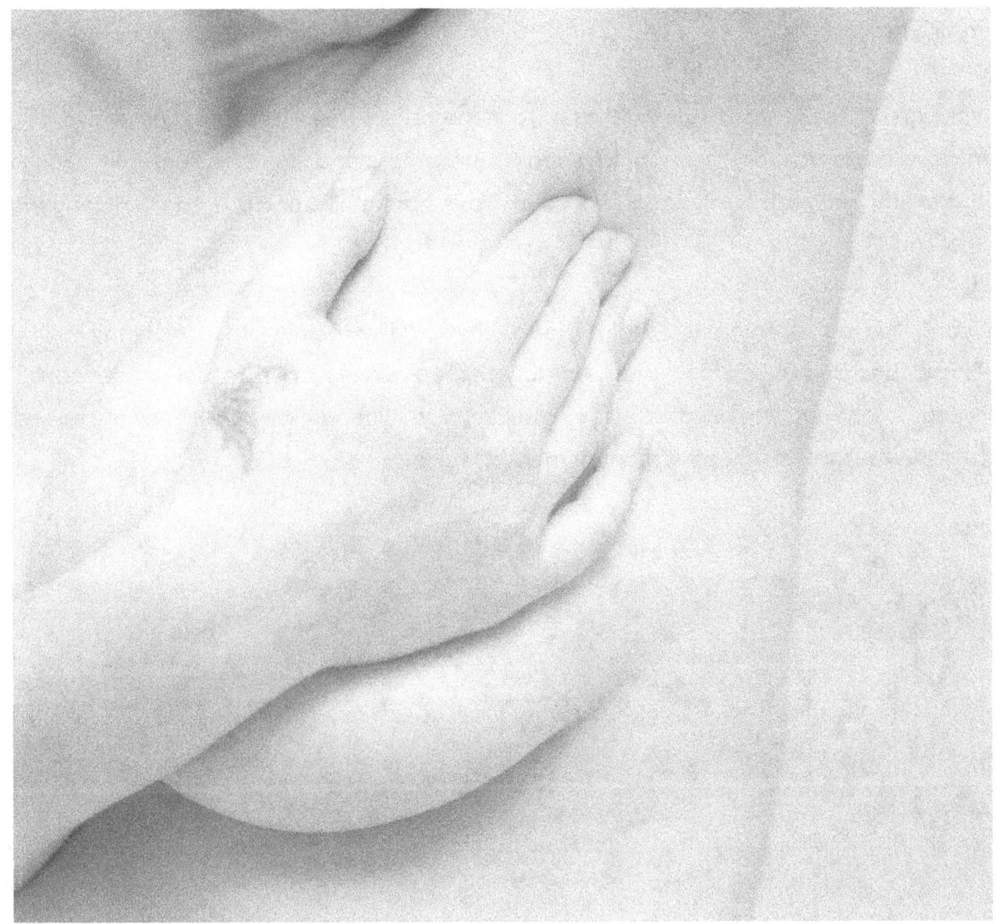

Many of my patients in the clinic have been treated for their Breast Cancer many years prior. For some of these women, the absence of scar tissue treatment has led to years of chronic pain. The best news I can share with you is that even older scar tissue can respond to current Physiotherapy techniques. I genuinely hope that it is encouraging to read that I have successfully treated women who had Breast Cancer 5, 10, 15 and even 20 years prior. I have been able to provide pain relief on at least some level for all of these women. Just because you may not have experienced treatment earlier does not mean there is no role for treatment now.

The significance of scar tissue extends beyond the visible. These remnants can evolve into sources of pain or discomfort, impeding movement and even skin sensitivity. Such scars may react adversely to light touch such as from clothing or a bra, compounding the challenge.

Scar tissue management is a realm where the expertise of physiotherapists shines. These specialist Physiotherapists, notably those experienced in breast cancer care, recognize the nuances of various scars resulting from different surgeries. They are poised to guide you through effective management strategies.

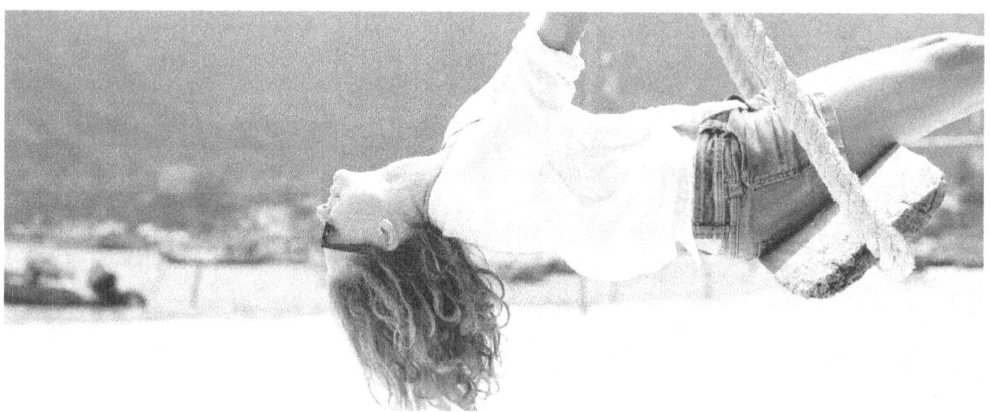

In addressing scar tissue, simple techniques come into play including education on how you can perform your own self massage. Massage often assumes a central role. Patients are empowered with knowledge on self-massaging their scar tissue, fostering a sense of ownership in their recovery journey. This therapeutic touch, combined with stretching and specialised products, such as Mobiderm® or Comfiwave®, enhances mobility and reduces scar-related discomfort.

Your healing journey is infused with the direction and assistance of experts skilled in navigating the difficulties of scar tissue. You can overcome the challenges of scar care by collaborating with a trained physiotherapist and adopting a road of recovery and comfort.

05 Unveiling Radiation Fibrosis Scarring

Moving on to radiation fibrosis scarring, a frequently overlooked side effect of breast cancer treatment. This topic is particularly close to my heart, as its under-discussion has spurred my passion to raise awareness.

After undergoing a lumpectomy, many women undergo radiation therapy, a common path in breast cancer treatment. Although, many women who undergo mastectomy may also require radiation to their chest wall. What's often not discussed at the time of treatment is the delayed side effects of radiation.

My clinic frequently involves women seeking help weeks, months, or even years post-radiation and lumpectomy or mastectomy. They grapple with persistent breast pain or chest wall discomfort. This distress is often attributed to the impact of radiation, causing tightening and thickening in the radiated area.

Imagine everyday tasks becoming trying endeavours-raising your arm, hanging laundry, or simply moving-all accompanied by tightness, soreness, and tenderness. While any unusual changes in the chest wall should be addressed with your medical team, it's important to note that a collection of symptoms and are common after radiation. This may include breast pain, breast swelling, breast shrinkage, and sudden onset of restricted shoulder range of movement.

In my practice, treating breast pain is a regular occurrence, frequently arising after both surgery and radiation. Simple yet effective methods come into play-massage, scar tissue release, and applying products like Mobiderm, Medi Lymph Pads or Comfiwave®.

If you are struggling with prolonged breast pain or chest wall discomfort post-radiation ask your General Practitioner or Medical Team for a referral to a Lymphoedema therapist who is experienced in treating Radiation Fibrosis. Take solace in knowing that while this experience is common, in the majority of cases appropriate treatment techniques can significantly improve symptoms. For many women, pain-free living after breast cancer treatment is attainable, as long as it's addressed with the appropriate care and expertise.

06 Fortifying Against Osteoporosis

Turning our attention to an often-overlooked aspect of breast cancer recovery, we uncover the issue of osteoporosis (also known as low bone mineral density). For some women following Breast Cancer, this topic can be under-addressed. However, knowledge is your greatest defence, prevention is key and knowing your treatment options is incredibly valuable.

A wise first step in preventing osteoporosis is figuring out your baseline bone mineral density. You may have previously had a bone mineral density test that showed you had osteopenia or osteoporosis, both of which are bone-thinning conditions.

Mainly, osteoporosis denotes severe bone thinning, while osteopenia is its predecessor and denotes less severe thinning.

But here's the beacon of hope: Bone mineral density can be improved. Engaging in resistance training, adopting appropriate supplements and medications, and embracing sunlight exposure and vitamin D can fortify your bone stock. **Remarkably, numerous women have bolstered their bone mineral density, establishing a healthier foundation.**

A pivotal concern lies in breast cancer treatment's effect on bone health. Postmenopausal women and those who have undergone chemotherapy face double the risk of osteoporosis compared to the general population. Further to this, some hormone-blocking medications used to treat oestrogen-positive Breast Cancers can also significantly reduce bone mineral density. This underscores the importance of proactively addressing this risk.

A lurking danger of undetected osteoporosis lies in the potential for fractures resulting from falls. Preventing such an ordeal is a priority worth pursuing. To this end, consult your medical team-your surgeon, oncologist, or GP-and arrange a bone mineral density test. With this baseline knowledge, you can take the necessary steps to safeguard your bone health.

Should you discover a diminished bone mineral density or wish to stave off osteoporosis proactively, consider enlisting the expertise of a specialized physiotherapist or exercise physiologist well-versed in breast cancer care. They can tailor a resistance training regimen (also known as strength training): a potent weapon against osteoporosis. Remember, a resilient skeleton is not just a goal; it's a tangible reality within reach.

07 Navigating Lymphoedema Management

As we progress, we confront the critical subject of lymphoedema. For many women, this term enters their vocabulary early in their breast cancer journey. As we've highlighted, lymphoedema emerges as a common aftermath of breast cancer treatment, particularly when lymph nodes are removed from the armpit or the arm or when radiation targets the chest wall or armpit.

Lymphoedema, characterized by chronic progressive swelling of the upper limb, can also extend to the breast and chest wall. Addressing this concern constitutes a central focus for physiotherapists skilled in Lymphoedema and breast cancer care.

Among the arsenal of treatments, exercise programs tailored to enhance lymphatic flow, manual lymphatic drainage, and self-lymphatic drainage play pivotal roles. Equipping patients with techniques for self-massage to alleviate excess lymphatic fluid becomes a cornerstone. Compression garments, revered as a gold standard in lymphoedema management and prevention, are not to be overlooked.

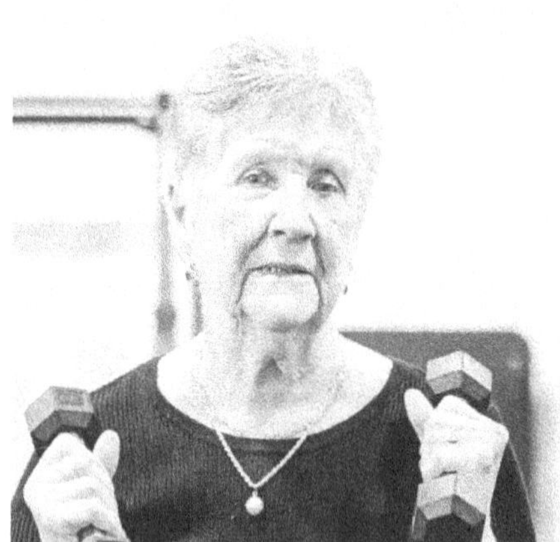
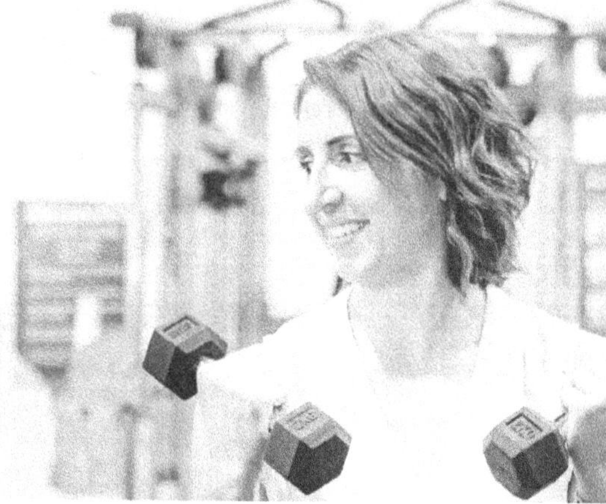

www.BreastCancerRevolution.co

Recall the counsel from our earlier discussion: securing a pre-operative L-Dex score – a gauge of lymphatic status-emerges as a potent preventive measure. But should this not materialize, obtaining a post-operative L-Dex score swiftly after surgery is a pragmatic alternative. The diligent oversight of specialized physiotherapists, occupational therapists, or nurses experienced in lymphoedema care proves indispensable during the chemotherapy and radiation phases.

Lymphoedema, and its management calls for a number of proactive measures. Each step in the process holds profound significance, from prevention to early detection and proficient management. Your commitment to thwarting or mitigating its impact will significantly influence your journey toward recovery.

08 Revitalizing Sexual Health

Let's shed light on a subject that has been veiled in secrecy for far too long: sexual health after Breast Cancer. Surprisingly and sadly, the conversation surrounding this issue is still gravely underdeveloped for women coping with the effects of breast cancer. Even more depressingly, research shows that healthcare providers frequently fail to address patients' sexual health and well-being. Medical and Allied Health Professionals need to ask their Breast Cancer patients about the impact of Breast Cancer treatment on their sexual health and provide referrals, where appropriate and required, to Women's Health Physiotherapists and Sexual Therapists.

We must courageously confront the realities and shed light on the myriad of solutions available to enhance sexual health and well-being post-breast cancer. Collaborating with dedicated Women's Health physiotherapists in my clinic, I continually witness the transformative impact of addressing this issue head-on.

Countless women approach me, grappling with various challenges stemming from breast cancer such as vaginal dryness, diminished libido, discomfort during intercourse, and the psychological toll it exacts to name but a few examples.

Let's be clear: sexual health encompasses not just physical factors but also mental and emotional elements. In many instances, sexual therapists, psychologists and counsellors prove invaluable allies in this journey. The path forward is not always easy, but working with the right Health Professionals in a supportive, safe environment can significantly improve the circumstances, no matter what aspect of your sexual health has been affected. I have witnessed many women make phenomenal recoveries by engaging with Women's Health Physiotherapists particularly.

Whether you're in a relationship or navigating this journey independently, take heart-a network of support is ready to guide you. Reach out, and I can connect you with the experts who specialize in improving sexual health post-breast cancer. Remember, you're far from alone in this experience, and a wealth of resources awaits to empower you in reclaiming your sexual well-being after breast cancer.

09 Overcoming Fatigue

I want to discuss the challenges of dealing with fatigue—a very common side effect when traversing the terrains of breast cancer treatment. Whether you're undergoing chemotherapy, radiation, or hormone therapy, fatigue often takes centre stage as a persistent symptom. A surprising revelation: exercise is a potent antidote to combat this weariness. This paradoxical solution may sound counterintuitive, but it holds immense promise.

When confronting fatigue, the guidance of a seasoned physiotherapist or exercise physiologist specializing in breast cancer becomes invaluable. These experts balance boosting your energy and ensuring the exercise regimen aligns with your unique circumstances. In other words-an experienced Health Professional will tailor your exercise program by taking into consideration all factors about your current treatment, medical history, and personal circumstances.

Indeed, fatigue is a familiar foe throughout your journey, but exercise can emerge as a amazing ally. Particularly when it comes to combating side effects such as brain fog, which can impact all corners of your life if left untreated. Exercise may not seem the appropriate antidote when all you want to do is lie down and rest, but the highest standards of research back exercise all the way when it comes to treating the side effects of Breast Cancer.

COSA (Clinical Oncology Society of Australia) offers a wealth of insight through its comprehensive Position Statements on exercise and cancer, spanning over a decade. These documents champion exercise as a powerful tool to combat fatigue during cancer treatment (Cormie et al, 2018).

Remember, your exercise program should be tailored to your chemotherapy, radiation, and beyond treatment phase. Seek a local physiotherapist or exercise physiologist versed in breast cancer care; they'll collaborate with you to design an exercise regimen that complements your treatment path. Rest assured, embracing exercise doesn't mean forsaking rest – both are vital components of your recovery journey. Also remember that if local Health Professionals are not available in your area, Telehealth appointments can be extremely beneficial.

10 Regaining Strength: Overcoming Muscle Atrophy

Let's shine a light on the subject of physical deconditioning, a subject sometimes overshadowed by the difficulties of treating breast cancer. This is another significant side effect of Breast Cancer treatment that is very under-addressed. It's amazing how quickly muscle mass and strength can deteriorate throughout procedures and treatments, especially in the affected arm on the side of the body that is being treated.

Post-surgery, muscle mass, and strength loss can take many by surprise. Even simple tasks like lifting a grandchild, carrying groceries, or hanging out washing may feel difficult. The solution lies in a tailored exercise regimen designed to rebuild strength in key areas: the shoulder, neck, upper back, and chest wall.

Notably, significant loss of muscle mass can also occur in the lower body. Consider how much your usual routine may have been affected since diagnosis: your active treatment typically requires many hours of driving to and from appointments, sitting in waiting rooms, sitting and talking with Medical Professionals, sitting or lying down for treatment or procedures, and increased periods of rest. None of the above requires the lower body to be utilized and hence muscle wastage in the legs can be profound.

Protecting the chest wall, often an instinctive response, inadvertently leads to muscle loss. Shielding an area can restrict movement, impair posture, and limit arm use. To counteract this, engaging with exercise professionals well-versed in breast cancer care is essential-physiotherapists and exercise physiologists. They are adept at crafting programs that target muscle revival post-surgery, chemotherapy, and radiation.

The benefits of regaining strength extend beyond the physical. A restored sense of strength transcends into improved self-esteem and mental well-being.

Often, emotional aspects interplay with the physical, given the emotional toll of breast cancer journeys. Exercise releases endorphins, our "happy hormones" that make us feel better emotionally and is one of the most effective weapons against poor mental and emotional health during and after Breast Cancer.

Why start down this road of muscle strength restoration? Because the gains go beyond the physical. Increased strength helps prevent lymphoedema, boosts energy levels, enhances body image and fosters increased self-confidence. Exercise is a powerful therapeutic tool that improves short-term quality of life during treatment and overall well-being. By embracing fitness, you're actively moving toward a stronger, healthier, and more independent future.

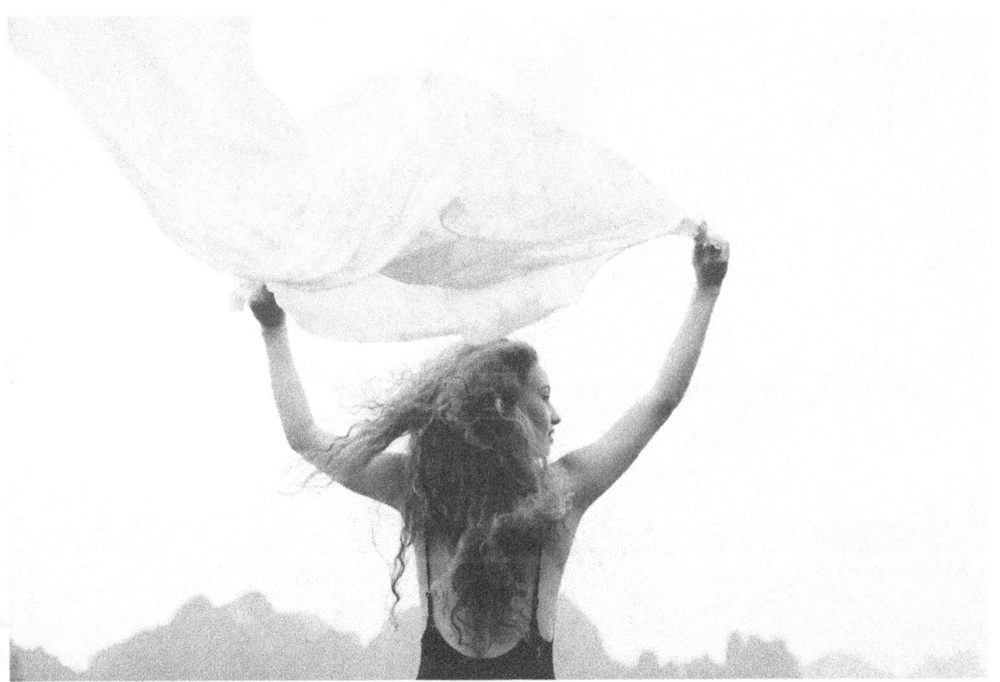

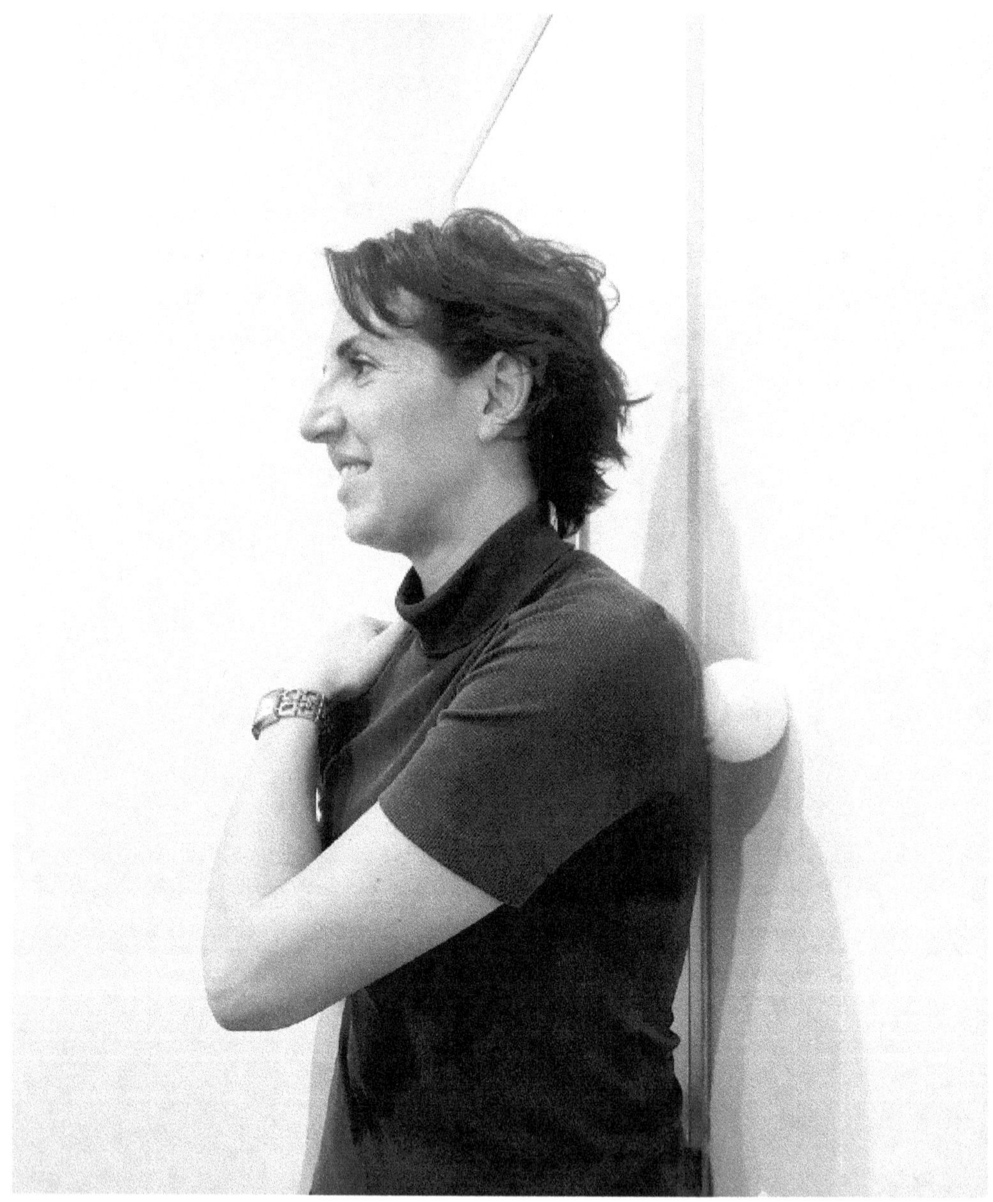

1.2 The Importance of an Early Physiotherapy Appointment

I want to now emphasize why making that first physiotherapy consultation soon after receiving a breast cancer diagnosis is so important. The importance of that first session cannot be overstated, even though it may not be common practice to refer patients to physiotherapy right away. Aiming for an appointment within the first two to four weeks following a diagnosis or surgery is so beneficial for so many reasons. As mentioned previously, and in an ideal situation, every woman would be referred for a pre-surgical baseline L-Dex Test.

The advantages of early involvement with a physiotherapist cannot be overstated, even if surgery is delayed and chemotherapy is the initial course of treatment (neo-adjuvant chemotherapy). This chapter clarifies the importance of an initial Physiotherapy appointment in addressing many of the overlooked side effects of breast cancer treatment.

Reason 1: Shoulder Range of Motion

One of the primary purposes of this initial visit to physiotherapy is to evaluate and treat any potential limitations in the shoulder range of motion. Limited mobility in the shoulder area after surgery is typical due to cording, surgical scars, discomfort, and protective behaviours.

It's interesting to note that patients may mistakenly assume they have fully recovered their shoulder range while, in reality, they are still missing the final 10 to 20 degrees. **Here** is when a specialized physiotherapist's knowledge is so valuable. They can recognize these differences and create specialized therapies to deal with persistent tension or stiffness problems.

Commonly, patients are not told when to discontinue their post-operative exercises. I'm specifically referring here to the exercises typically provided in most hospitals following breast surgery. If progressing to full shoulder range of motion stalls, and complete shoulder mobility remains elusive beyond approximately 4 weeks post-surgery, it could indicate underlying issues beyond the immediate surgical aftermath – such as tight muscles or other sources of discomfort.

If radiation therapy is part of the treatment plan, regaining full shoulder range of motion is crucial for positioning during radiation treatment. I have seen many women struggle through the weeks of radiation treatment if their shoulder range is restricted. Early Physiotherapy to address any limitations in shoulder mobility are vital to reduce issues later on during radiation treatment.

We all need a functional range of movement in our shoulders to perform daily activities like lifting and carrying. It doesn't matter if you are in your late 30s or early 80s when you're diagnosed with Breast Cancer when it comes to addressing shoulder mobility. Women of all ages are performing tasks every day that require optimal shoulder mobility without pain or restriction.

Reason 2: Addressing Ongoing Pain

Addressing and managing persistent pain is another vital reason to access physiotherapy as soon as possible after Breast Cancer surgery or other treatments.

Many side effects of Breast Cancer treatment can contribute to ongoing pain and discomfort, highlighting the necessity of a physiotherapist's involvement. For instance, cording often involves pain and restricted mobility. Trapped fluids like seromas or general post-surgical swelling may be uncomfortable and restrict shoulder mobility. As highlighted earlier, the inclination to protect the chest wall or breast can inadvertently create tension and weakness which in turn exacerbates pain.

The phenomenon of post-operative myalgia, where the nervous system heightens pain sensitivity, can further complicate matters. In such instances, the guidance and interventions provided by a physiotherapist can play a pivotal role in pain resolution. Addressing pain is not only paramount for restoring physical function but also for mental well-being. If pain is uncontrolled, undiagnosed and untreated, it can quickly affect many areas of your life, including your emotional health.

Chronic pain can significantly reduce motivation to engage in activities like exercise or adopt a balanced diet during breast cancer treatment. Neglecting pain management could lead to a cascade of effects, particularly your sleep quality and quantity. By proactively seeking pain relief through physiotherapy, individuals can significantly enhance their overall well-being and quality of life as they navigate their breast cancer journey.

Reason 3: Preventing Lymphoedema

One of the pivotal reasons to promptly engage with a physiotherapist after receiving a breast cancer diagnosis is to proactively work on preventing lymphoedema. Lymphoedema is a potential consequence stemming from surgical removal of lymph nodes or radiation of lymph nodes or lymph vessels. This condition results in the accumulation of excessive lymphatic fluid in the arm, chest wall or breast.

Individuals diagnosed with breast cancer are particularly susceptible to lymphoedema. The risk is present whether you undergo full axillary lymph node dissection (more than four lymph nodes removed) or a sentinel node biopsy (typically between one and four). Your risk is lower if you've only had a sentinel node biopsy, but there is still a risk of developing lymphoedema.

It is crucial to dispel misconceptions about lymphoedema risk, otherwise, some women who have only had a sentinel node biopsy may not be referred for lymphoedema screening and prevention education.

Educating yourself about lymphoedema is key, and rather than succumbing to fear, empowering yourself through awareness is by far the best approach. By staying informed, you become alert to the precautions and actions that can reduce your risk of developing lymphoedema. Myths and misconceptions surrounding lymphoedema abound in the community, emphasizing the importance of seeking accurate information from credible sources.

For instance, concerns about using your affected arm more frequently and potentially triggering lymphoedema is misinformation. Regularly engaging your arm promotes muscle contractions and physical movement that enhance lymphatic flow. The lymphatic system relies on muscle activity, gravity, and motion to facilitate fluid drainage, making regular arm usage a positive practice.

Additionally, advancements in healthcare have introduced tools like L-Dex measuring devices. Physical therapists, physiotherapists, occupational therapists, and specially trained nurses can access these devices. L-Dex devices offer an early snapshot of your lymphatic system's condition, facilitating proactive intervention by detecting signs of lymphoedema at its earliest stage.

Incorporating these preventive measures into your breast cancer journey can significantly reduce the likelihood of developing lymphoedema, granting you greater control and confidence throughout your treatment and recovery process. By partnering with a physiotherapist who specializes in lymphoedema, you are better equipped to navigate the complexities of lymphoedema prevention and ensure the best possible outcomes for your well-being.

Reason 4: Exercise Guidance

An additional compelling reason to prioritize a physiotherapy consultation after receiving a breast cancer diagnosis is to gain valuable exercise education. Exercise emerges as a cornerstone of navigating the challenges posed by breast cancer treatment. The benefits of engaging in regular physical activity extend beyond the physical realm to encompass significant improvements in mental and emotional health. Integrating exercise into your routine can also mitigate the side effects of various breast cancer treatments.

Amid the spectrum of breast cancer treatments, chemotherapy often brings forth debilitating side effects like nausea and fatigue. Remarkably, consistent and moderate exercise has been proven to alleviate these distressing symptoms substantially. It's essential to recognize that exercise doesn't necessitate training for a marathon; even light and manageable physical activity can yield remarkable benefits. Further to this, chemotherapy has been shown to accelerate muscle mass loss, making exercise imperative in reducing the impact of chemotherapy, and recovering from it, after Breast Cancer treatment.

However, what truly sets the stage for successful exercise integration is learning to perform it appropriately. This is where the expertise of a Physiotherapist or Exercise Physiologist becomes invaluable. Many women frequently ask me this question, including Medical and Health Professionals diagnosed with Breast Cancer that I have cared for: what is the safest and most effective way to exercise during my breast cancer journey? So even trained Health Professionals can be very unsure of how to safely commence exercise following their diagnosis. In this regard, breast cancer presents a unique context that requires tailored guidance to ensure safety, efficacy, and comfort.

Addressing fatigue constitutes a pivotal challenge during breast cancer treatment, often leaving individuals drained and apprehensive about engaging in physical activity. Paradoxically, research consistently highlights the positive impact of exercise on fatigue management. By adhering to proper exercise protocols under the supervision of a physical therapist, physiotherapist, or exercise physiologist, individuals can experience remarkable alleviation of fatigue and an overall enhancement of well-being.

Incorporating exercise into your breast cancer journey requires a delicate balance between staying active and tailoring your exercise that is appropriate for each different treatment phase and how you are responding to it. The specialized knowledge of physiotherapists equips them to provide you with tailored exercise plans that consider your unique circumstances and treatment stage. This may include factors like how you are coping with your current chemotherapy regime, or at what point you can recommence strength training after surgery. Navigating the complexities of exercise during breast cancer treatment necessitates expert guidance, which can be safely and effectively prescribed through a Physiotherapy or Exercise Physiology consultation.

In conclusion, by embracing exercise as a powerful ally in your breast cancer journey and seeking guidance from a knowledgeable Physiotherapist, you pave the way for improved physical and mental well-being, effectively counteracting treatment challenges.

When prescribing exercises, it would be ideal if the Health Professional you're working with is experienced in treating breast cancer patients and survivors. As I previously mentioned, just one physiotherapy appointment is crucial in the first two to four weeks.

Don't despair if this window has passed - you can still benefit from seeking a Physiotherapist even years after your Breast Cancer treatment. As an experienced Breast Cancer Physiotherapist, I firmly believe that my role with all of my Breast Cancer patients or survivors is to facilitate a supportive and education-rich environment from active treatment to the years beyond so that you can start to get your life back after one of the most challenging journeys a woman can face.

BREAST CANCER REVOLUTION

Jen McKenzie

Remember to access your goodies in the
BCR Resource Vault.
Scan the QR code above to Access.

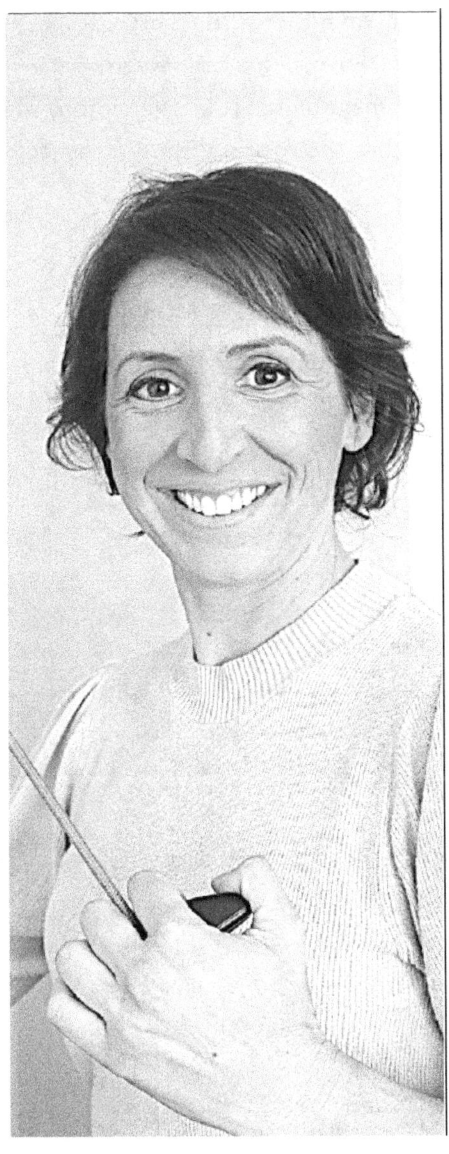

Embracing Freedom:

Range of Movement
Exercises for Enhanced
Recovery after Breast
Cancer Surgery

In this chapter, we delve into a crucial aspect of your journey to recovery after breast cancer surgery: range of movement exercises. If you've recently emerged from breast cancer surgery, you might be feeling tight and sore. However, fear not; as you tackle these exercises, you'll gradually regain function and mobility. Let's explore this essential range of movement exercises tailored for post-breast cancer surgery recovery.

01 Shoulder Range of Motion

First, let's discuss why it's imperative to regain mobility after breast cancer surgery, starting with restoring the shoulder range of motion. Following a lumpectomy or mastectomy, many individuals instinctively protect the affected side, even if they're unaware of it. This protective response can lead to limited shoulder use. Early movement is crucial to restoring arm function.

By initiating movement early, you can help prevent conditions like frozen shoulder (adhesive capsulitis) or bursitis, which often develop when you neglect shoulder mobility. Another compelling reason to start moving your shoulder early is to reduce the risk of lymphedema. Contrary to common misconceptions, moving your arm frequently promotes lymphatic flow, potentially reducing the risk of lymphedema rather than triggering it. Embrace movement; it's beneficial for your lymphatic system.

02 Avoid Stiff Joints

Beyond the shoulders, it's essential to prevent other joints around the surgical area from stiffening. Keep your elbow, wrist, hand, fingers, neck, ribcage, and upper back mobile. Neglecting these areas can lead to discomfort and postural problems, which might come as a surprise to many.

Breast cancer surgery can impact your body's dynamics, even leading to issues like chest wall pain, headaches, breathing restrictions or tension down your arm.

Therefore, conscious movement is key to maintaining overall joint and muscle health during your recovery.

03 Increase Blood Flow

Boosting blood flow plays a pivotal role in the healing process. Blood flow is a driving force behind scar tissue healing and soft tissue recovery post-surgery. Movement enhances blood circulation, ultimately aiding in your healing journey.

Additionally, regular movement fosters confidence. Many individuals fear moving their arms due to concerns about lymphedema. However, the lymphatic system has no major pump of its own which in turn means it relies on muscle contraction and movement to shift lymphatic fluid. Confidence in your body's capabilities grows as you realize the benefits of movement.

Reducing the fear surrounding movement after breast cancer surgery is crucial. Early engagement in functional movements minimizes the risk of long-term dysfunction.

04 Avoid Cording

Another motivation to initiate early movement is to prevent a condition known as cording or axillary web syndrome. Cording presents as thick, cord-like structures in the armpit, possibly extending down the arm. From my clinical experience, I believe cording to be significant to extreme nerve tension. Cording initially occurs due to trauma from surgical interventions in the armpit, such as lymph node removal.

Treatment is targeted with gentle but specific nerve stretches to start resolving the cording. Frequency, repetition and achieving a tolerable stretch on the nerve are important aspects of these exercises.

04 Avoid Cording

Aim for three sessions a day, with around 20 repetitions of each exercise. However, adjust according to your comfort level, as each person's progress is unique.

The nerve mobilisation stretches require a specific technique which can be best viewed on my YouTube Channel 'The Breast Cancer Physio'

Post-Surgery Range of Motion Exercises

We'll now discuss the frequency and repetitions of these exercises. Aim for three sessions daily, but remember, overdoing or underdoing it isn't beneficial. Listen to your body and adjust as needed. You'll experience significant changes in the first few weeks post-surgery, so take it easy.

Each exercise should involve around 20 repetitions. However, this can vary between individuals. Pay attention to your body, especially if certain movements feel more painful than others.

Here are the following exercises:

Wrist Movements: Start with flexion-extension (moving the wrist back and forth) and rotation (twisting movement). You can perform these on both sides, even if only one side underwent surgery.

Finger Movements: Open and close your fist, ensuring all fingers move. Test your dexterity by touching each finger to your thumb in a movement called opposition.

Elbow Movements: Flex and extend (bend and straighten) your elbow as much as you're comfortable with, particularly in the initial days.

Shoulder Movements: Roll your shoulders gently to relax them and prevent stiffness. Gradually lift your affected arm, clasping your fingers together, and raise it to a comfortable level. Don't push yourself too hard, only go as far as you can tolerate.

Rib cage and Upper Back Exercise: Deliberately slump and then extend your upper body. This exercise reveals any tightness in your back and reminds you of the ideal posture to aim for.

Neck Movements: Turn your neck left and right, tilt it left and right, and move it backward and forward. Do these movements three times a day in each direction to prevent neck stiffness.

Nerve Stretching Exercise: This exercise involves a combined movement of the elbow joint and the wrist to stretch the nerves gently, potentially preventing cording. Extend your elbow and wrist back and forth without raising your shoulder too high.

Walking Fingers Up the Wall: Crawl your fingers up a wall, then slide them back down. This exercise provides support for your shoulder joint and measures your progress as you get higher.

Remember not to remove your hands from the wall while coming back down, especially if your shoulder is weak.

Lastly, if you experience severe or worsening pain during these exercises or sense something isn't right, consult your medical team.

Post-operative conditions like seroma, infection, hematoma, or DVT can occur. Timely communication with your healthcare providers is essential.

Many women present in my clinic 6 months following their surgery still trying to perform the post-surgical exercises. Now, you might be wondering when to discontinue these exercises. While it varies from person to person, stopping around two to three weeks after surgery is common if you're progressing well. From my clinical experience, if you are still experiencing restriction with any of the post-operative exercises beyond 3-4 weeks, you need to seek a Physiotherapy assessment.

However, if you struggle with specific movements, such as raising your arm overhead or notice cording or tension around your rib cage, it's time to consult a physiotherapist who specialises in breast cancer. They can help you regain mobility and alleviate pain. Many women present in my clinic 6 months following their surgery still doing the post-surgical exercises. If you can perform the full range of movement, these exercises are not particularly useful. If you still cannot perform movement without restriction, these post-operative exercises won't be the answer to resolving the issue.

Moreover, as your range of motion improves, you can transition to a resistance exercise program, typically around four weeks post-surgery, provided there are no complications like infection or unstable seromas. Keep in mind that some exercises may need to continue longer if certain movements remain challenging.

In summary, these range-of-motion exercises are essential for your recovery and long-term well-being. Adjust them to your comfort level, stay patient, and consult your medical team if you encounter any issues. Remember, your healing journey is unique, and these exercises can pave the way for a healthier, more mobile future.

BREAST CANCER REVOLUTION

Jen McKenzie

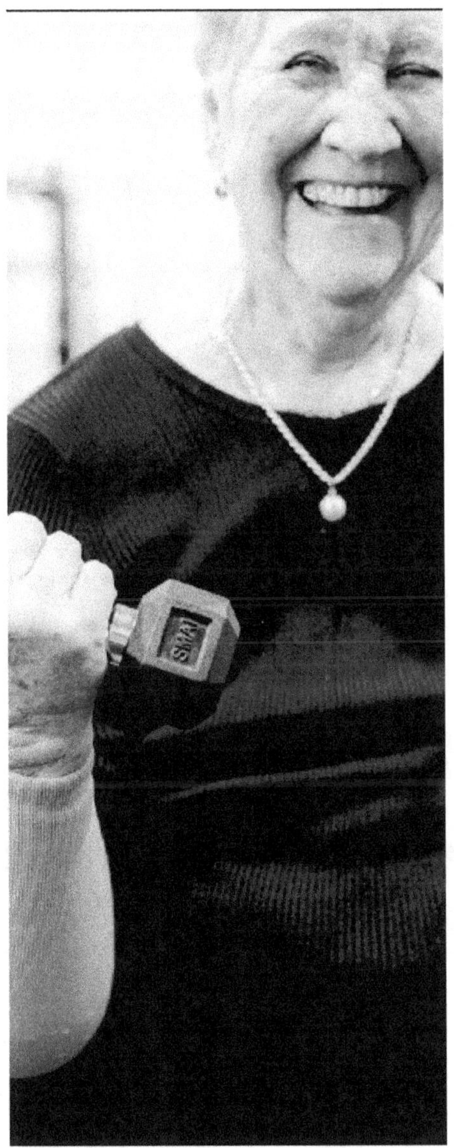

Understanding Lymphoedema:

Recognizing, Preventing, and Addressing the Impact

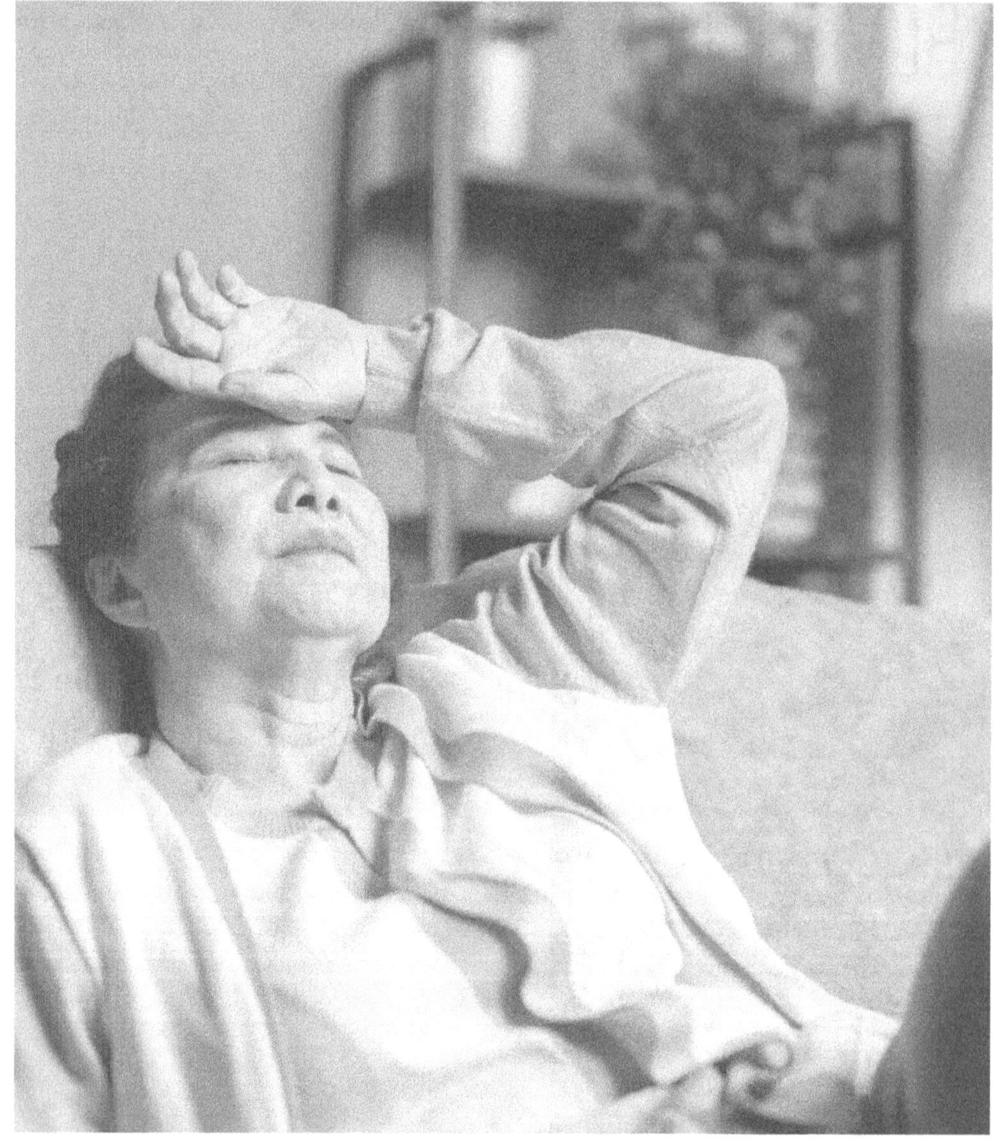

3.1 Signs and Symptoms of Lymphoedema

If you're navigating the challenges of breast cancer, it's essential to remain proactive in safeguarding your mental, physical, and emotional well-being. Lymphoedema is one of the nastier potential side effects of Breast Cancer and it can be overwhelming just to be at risk of this condition, let alone be diagnosed with lymphoedema. In this section, I'll explore the signs and symptoms of lymphoedema, a possible consequence of breast cancer treatment, following lymph node removal in the armpit or radiation have been performed.

Symptom 1: Swelling

Lymphoedema is often misunderstood as a sudden ballooning of the affected limb, but this misconception can lead to delayed detection. In reality, the early stages of lymphoedema are more subtle and may be felt before they are seen. Recognizing these early signs is crucial for individuals who have undergone breast cancer treatment or are at risk of lymphoedema.

Intermittent and Mild Swelling: Lymphoedema can manifest as mild, intermittent, or fluctuating swelling. It doesn't always engulf the entire arm; it can appear as a localized patch of swelling.

Inside of the Elbow: A significant indicator of lymphoedema is puffiness on the inside of the elbow. This is often one of the earliest signs, so pay close attention to any puffiness you notice, whether seen or felt.

Indentations: Watch out for unexpected indentations left by jewellery, clothing, or watches. If an item you regularly wear suddenly leaves a mark that wasn't there before, it's a signal worth investigating.

Changes in Bony Structures: Another sign to be aware of is the disappearance of bony bumps along the knuckles, wrist, or elbow. If these noticeable landmarks become less apparent or disappear, it may indicate swelling.

Self-Examination: When examining your arm, locate these bony bumps. If you can't find them around your wrist or elbow, it's a potential sign of swelling.

Remember, we often sense or feel swelling before it becomes visually apparent. If you experience intermittent or fluctuating swelling, don't hesitate to seek professional evaluation, especially if you are at risk of lymphoedema.

Seeking Professional Guidance: Consulting a qualified physiotherapist, nurse or occupational therapist specializing in lymphoedema is paramount for individuals who have undergone breast cancer treatment and are at risk of lymphoedema. These health professionals can provide a comprehensive assessment and guidance tailored to your needs. Remember to consider linking in with a Lymphoedema Therapist via Telehealth if there is not one available in your local area

Symptom 2: Heaviness

Heaviness is a sensation that can indicate lymphoedema and is essential to recognize for those who have undergone breast cancer treatment or are at risk. It can be described as the arm feeling heavier, similar to the sensation of a "dead-arm punch". Imagine the feeling of your arm being noticeably heavier than it typically is when held by your side. This sensation can occur alongside or independent of visible swelling.

If you experience this uncharacteristic heaviness, especially when coupled with swelling or other potential lymphoedema symptoms, it is crucial to seek professional evaluation promptly.

Symptom 3: Tightness

Another significant symptom to be mindful of is the sensation of tightness in the affected arm. This sensation can be likened to the feeling that the skin around your arm is constricting, causing discomfort. Tightness in the arm can manifest and feel as if the skin is too snug for the underlying structures. This sensation might extend along the entire length of the arm. If you experience the sensation of tightness in your arm, it is advisable to seek a professional assessment promptly, especially if other potential lymphoedema symptoms are present.

Symptom 4: Pins and Needles

While not the most frequently observed symptom in my experience when diagnosing lymphoedema, the sensation of "pins and needles" occurs occasionally. This tingling sensation is typically described as a diffuse tingling that courses through the limb rather than being concentrated in specific areas. While variations in the presentation of "pins and needles" may exist, this is the classic description I've encountered in my practice.

Distinguishing from Peripheral Neuropathy: It's important to note that when we mention "pins and needles" in the context of lymphoedema, we are not referring to the common side effect of chemotherapy known as peripheral neuropathy. Peripheral neuropathy typically affects the tips of the fingers or toes and tends to occur simultaneously on both sides of the body. In contrast, lymphoedema often manifests in one arm making bilateral upper-limb lymphoedema uncommon.

If you are experiencing tingling sensations primarily in your fingertips and it affects both sides of your body, it is more likely related to peripheral neuropathy associated with chemotherapy. However, if you remain uncertain about your symptoms, I strongly encourage you to seek a local physiotherapist specializing in lymphoedema. They can provide a comprehensive evaluation and appropriate diagnosis.

Symptom 5: Ache

When we refer to the "ache" symptom, it's important to clarify that we're not discussing an intense or severe type of pain. In my experience, very few patients with lymphoedema report significant pain. While it may occur occasionally, the ache associated with lymphoedema is described as a dull discomfort akin to a persistent, low-level toothache rather than excruciating pain.

More often than not, if patients experience pain they will often report their hand being painful. I suspect this is due to the fact that there is not much room for extra fluid to reside in the hand as there are so many bones, ligaments and tendons taking up the majority of the space.

Extra fluid in the hand places mechanical pressure on these tissue structures and thus pain is noticed sooner than other parts of the arm.

If you are experiencing severe pain in conjunction with swelling, it's advisable to consider other potential causes beyond lymphoedema such as DVT (Deep Vein Thrombosis) or SVT (Superficial Vein Thrombosis). Such cases may warrant further investigations, such as a CT scan, Doppler ultrasound, or other diagnostic procedures to explore alternative medical conditions. Therefore, if you're encountering a mild, persistent ache in your arm, alongside any other signs or symptoms like swelling, heaviness, tightness, or pins and needles, I strongly recommend consulting your local physiotherapist for a thorough evaluation and diagnosis. If you are unable to access a trained Lymphoedema Therapist, I would advise touching base with your GP or Medical Team in the event pain is severe and persistent.

One crucial takeaway from this discussion is the importance of promptly addressing any suspicions or concerns related to lymphoedema's early signs and symptoms. Seeking assistance at the earliest possible stage offers the greatest opportunity to halt the progression of this condition toward a more advanced state.

It's worth noting that, excitingly, there have been instances where early onset lymphoedema has been successfully reversed. Yes, you read that correctly. However, this reversal is likely when lymphoedema is detected in its early phases. Should lymphoedema progress beyond this initial stage, the likelihood of complete reversal diminishes. Nonetheless, even if full reversal is not possible, early treatment can significantly enhance the manageability of the condition in the long run.

In essence, if you've received a lymphoedema diagnosis and it proves unresponsive to reversal efforts, you are still highly likely to experience a level of lymphoedema that is much more manageable with early, proactive intervention. Therefore, the best course of action is clear: do not procrastinate. Visit a Lymphoedema therapist promptly and request a comprehensive assessment to determine whether lymphoedema is the issue. Initiating intervention as early as possible affords you the greatest prospects for effectively managing or reversing this condition.

3.2 How Do I Know If I Have Lymphoedema?

Moving on to a crucial topic-how to determine whether you might have developed lymphoedema after undergoing breast cancer treatment. With the advancement of medical technology, we've come to understand that early-onset lymphoedema can manifest without overt symptoms.

Recognizing the Signs and Symptoms

There are five cardinal signs and symptoms of lymphoedema. These include:

• A sense of heaviness or tightness in the affected limb, specifically the "affected arm" (the arm that has undergone lymph node removal or radiation).
• Pins and needles sensation in the limb.
• A persistent, dull ache in the limb.
• Observable or palpable swelling in the limb.
• It's important to note that you may not experience all five symptoms at once; having just one or a combination of these signs is possible. However, these represent the classic indicators of lymphoedema emerging in a limb.

Crucially, there's the possibility of having none of these signs or symptoms while still having early-onset lymphoedema. This shouldn't cause undue concern. Instead, it underscores the significance of early diagnosis and intervention. The SOZO® is able to detect very early signs of fluid buildup in the upper limb. Hence you are diagnosing early onset lymphoedema when fluid levels are still very low. While lymphoedema might not yet be curable, advancements in medical technology provide hope for its resolution, especially during the early stages.

Challenging the Tape Measure Method

Traditionally, therapists have used tape measurements to diagnose lymphoedema, but I have reservations about this approach and research is certainly starting to back my concerns.

Measuring circumferences with tape doesn't account for variations in arm dominance, fatty tissue levels and muscle mass between individuals. Moreover, it assumes that any differences between limbs are due to fluid changes, which may not always be the case.

I understand that there may be differing opinions on this topic, but from my clinical experience, I avoid using tape measures for diagnosing lymphoedema unless it is absolutely necessary. The more comprehensive assessment offered by advanced medical technology, which I'll introduce shortly, offers a better alternative.

The Role of Early Diagnosis

Early diagnosis is crucial for effective lymphoedema management and potential resolution. Enter the ImpediMed SOZO® Digital Health Platform, a remarkable device that employs bioimpedance spectroscopy technology.

The SOZO is a user-friendly tool that involves a 30-second, pain-free test. It provides an L-DEX Score (Lymphoedema Index Score): a quick assessment that can help determine whether lymphoedema may be present. Importantly, it can also offer reassurance by confirming the absence of lymphoedema. Individuals with pacemakers, neurostimulators, or defibrillators should refrain from using this device due to contraindications. Portacaths and PICC lines, however, pose no issues.

Understanding SOZO's Capabilities

The SOZO device measures fluid, not lymphoedema or edema, precisely. It's highly sensitive to fluid changes and can detect even minor discrepancies between limbs, with a sensitivity allowing it to pick up small fluid variances.

It's worth noting that fluid may accumulate in the treated upper limb after breast surgery or radiation, causing swelling. This isn't necessarily lymphoedema but post-treatment edema. Therefore, it's crucial to interpret SOZO's results in the context of the patient's treatment timeline.

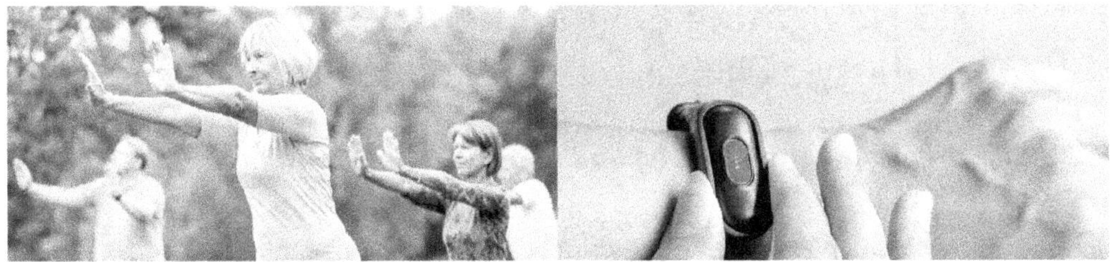

Monitoring with SOZO®

In cases where the L-DEX score suggests post-treatment swelling, close monitoring is essential. If the score remains elevated or continues to rise, early-onset lymphoedema is possible, and intervention becomes necessary. This intervention may include prescribing compression garments, teaching self-lymphatic drainage massage, and advising on skincare. The encouraging news is that early-onset lymphoedema can often be managed and potentially reversed with prompt intervention.

Leveraging Technology for Early Detection

The key takeaway is that if you're uncertain about early-onset lymphoedema, consider accessing the Impedimed SOZO® Digital Health Platform. While those in remote areas may have limited access, those in urban or regional centres can seek medical professionals who offer this service. If you are located in a remote region it is worth considering a trip to access a facility with a SOZO® device

The ImpediMed SOZO and its predecessor, the U400, can be instrumental in assessing L-DEX scores and monitoring for lymphoedema. I urge you to advocate for your healthcare team's support in locating practitioners with this technology, as early detection is pivotal in effectively managing or potentially resolving lymphoedema.

3.3 Navigating Environmental Factors and
Lifestyle Choices to Prevent Lymphoedema

01 Skin Care: Understanding the link to the Immune System

In understanding lymphoedema prevention, it's crucial to recognize that the lymphatic system plays a vital role in our immune defence. In fact, the Lymphatic System is part of the Immune System. If you've undergone lymph node removal due to breast cancer, the skin on the affected arm (the arm that has undergone lymph node removal or radiation) is compromised in terms of immunity. This impact on skin immunity is a lifelong change. Here's how you can protect it:

Regularly inspect the skin on the affected arm. Be vigilant for signs of infection, such as pain, redness, swelling, warmth, or pus. At the slightest suspicion of infection, seek immediate medical attention, preferably from your local GP, who can prescribe prophylactic antibiotics if an infection is indeed suspected.

The primary goal is to prevent the development of cellulitis, a broad skin infection that, when it progresses, could necessitate hospitalization and intravenous antibiotic treatment. Avoiding this scenario is essential, as cellulitis can trigger lymphoedema.

Moisturizing for Skin Integrity

Hydrating the skin is fundamental to maintaining its integrity and preventing skin breakdown. Daily moisturization is key, focusing on the arm where lymph nodes were removed or radiated. Choose water-based, low-pH creams that are less likely to cause skin irritation.

Brands such as Sorbolene are good options. Depending on which country you reside in will depend on what moisturisers are available. If unsure, ask your treating Medical Team or GP as to what moisturisers are safe to use, particularly during treatment. Always do a patch test to check for allergic reactions on your skin if you haven't used the product previously.

Stay hydrated from the inside out by drinking adequate amounts of fluid. Well-hydrated skin is more resilient, making it less prone to breakdown. Dry, wrinkly skin is much more likely to be at risk of infection.

02 Blood Pressure Measurements: Opt for the Unaffected Arm

If circumstances permit, it's advisable to utilize the arm that has not undergone lymph node removal or radiation for blood pressure measurements. This precaution minimizes potential risk of triggering lymphoedema.

While I haven't personally observed cases of lymphoedema onset immediately following a blood pressure test in my clinic, it's worth noting that documented instances exist in the medical literature where individuals suspect that a blood pressure cuff test may have triggered their lymphoedema. To err on the side of caution, if feasible, opt for the opposite arm—the one free from lymph node intervention.

Alternatively, you can explore the option of having a blood pressure cuff test administered around the ankle if avoiding the arms is your preference.

03: Needle Procedures: Pragmatic Guidance for Injections and Tests

When considering injections, vaccinations, and blood tests, my counsel remains consistent. If you possess an unaffected arm, it is preferable to use it.

However, it's essential to clarify that the primary concern does not revolve around the initial needle penetration, but rather the possibility of a needle stick injury, which can lead to complications such as bruising and inflammation at the site, which in turn may trigger lymphoedema. We discuss the risk of lymphoedema and the use of needles more in Section 3.4

Needle stick injuries typically occur when the needle cannot find a suitable vein or encounters unforeseen challenges. Therefore, if you find yourself in a situation where the use of an arm with prior lymph node intervention is necessary, we, as healthcare professionals, must take extra care to ensure that the procedure is as smooth as possible, reducing the likelihood of any injury or complications.

In the event of an unintentional procedure, such as a blood test on an arm with previous lymph node intervention, there's no immediate cause for alarm. However, it's prudent to monitor the arm for signs of swelling over the subsequent 24 to 48 hours. While there is a risk of infection resulting from the initial needle penetration, it is crucial to underscore that this risk is exceptionally low.

To reiterate the key takeaway: whenever possible, choose the arm untouched by lymph node procedures. In cases where interventions are deemed necessary on the affected arm, exercise caution to ensure a smooth and minimally invasive experience. For procedures like vaccinations and infusions that require extended time and fluid administration, consider the potential for additional strain on the lymphatic system in the affected arm. Exploring alternative options or utilizing the unaffected arm is advised.

If you are going into hospital for a procedure, you may need to have these discussions with your treating Surgeon and also your Anaesthetist. In recent years I have not only advised patients to discuss their requests with their Medical Team prior to surgery, but also to document their request to avoid Anaethetists using the affected arm during operations. Unfortunately there have been a number of cases where the patient's requests have been ignored.

04 Travel: Long Journeys and Lymphoedema

When embarking on extended journeys, particularly plane flights or car rides exceeding four hours, take precautions to prevent lymphoedema:

- Wear a properly fitted, appropriately graded compression sleeve on the affected arm to combat the stagnant nature of these activities. Remember-the lymphatic system has no pump of its own so stagnant activities can reduce lymphatic flow.
- Ensure that the compression sleeve is correctly fitted by a knowledgeable physiotherapist or occupational therapist experienced in breast cancer and lymphoedema care.
- If you are travelling by car or plane, wear the compression sleeve throughout the journey and for approximately one hour afterwards to promote healthy circulation.
- During prolonged periods of immobility, make an effort to move the at-risk limb regularly. This movement helps engage the muscle contractions around the lymphatics, aiding in the drainage of lymphatic fluid.

05 Climate Matters

Climate can have a significant impact on lymphoedema. In extreme temperatures, both hot and cold, you need to be vigilant. Let's explore these climate-related concerns.

Heat's Influence

High temperatures, especially in hot and humid climates, can trigger swelling in your limbs. The heat places added demands on your lymphatic system, making it work harder. To mitigate this risk, consider the following:

If possible, invest in air conditioning for your home to create a cool and comfortable environment.

• Avoid venturing outdoors during the hottest parts of the day.

• Avoid exercising in the hotter parts of the day unless in an air-conditioned space.

• Be cautious about prolonged exposure to intense heat sources such as thermal springs, jacuzzis, spas, saunas, and steam rooms. While it's essential to maintain your quality of life, be mindful of these activities, as excessive heat can overtax your lymphatic system.

The Cold Factor

On the flip side, extreme cold can also strain the lymphatic system. If you're heading to a frigid climate like snowy mountains or ski resorts, it's essential to bundle up and take extra precautions to protect limbs at risk of lymphoedema.

The key difference between heat and cold is that in cold environments, we are often more conscious of the need to protect ourselves. However, in persistently hot climates, finding relief can be a greater challenge. Therefore, it's crucial to have strategies in place to reduce your body heat during the warmer months.

Research whether your Government has any subsidies for electricity costs associated with medical conditions. Some Government rebate schemes allow subsidisation of electricity bills if you are suffering from conditions that are affected by heat, such as lymphoedema.

06 Body Composition Insights

Another crucial aspect to consider is your body composition. If you are overweight or obese your risk of developing lymphoedema is higher. Here's what you need to know:

Fatty tissue is a significant factor that can trigger lymphoedema, so if you fall into the overweight or obese category, working with a dietitian or exercise physiologist to reduce your body fat percentage can be highly beneficial.

Weight loss through a steady, healthy approach can dramatically lower your risk of lymphoedema or improve an existing condition.

Exercise Strategies

While exercise is essential for your overall well-being, it's crucial to approach it sensibly if you are at risk of or have lymphoedema. Suddenly commencing intense, high-volume physical activity can sometimes trigger lymphoedema, particularly if your system is deconditioned after a breast cancer experience. Here's what you should keep in mind:

Start Low, Progress Slow

Start low and progress slowly when resuming or initiating an exercise program. Avoid transitioning from minimal activity to an intense, seven-day workout regimen. This abrupt shift can increase the risk of lymphoedema. Consult a physiotherapist or exercise physiologist experienced in breast cancer and lymphoedema treatment. They can design an individualized exercise program tailored to your current fitness level, ensuring a gradual and safe progression.

07 Reduce risk of Sunburn

Protect yourself from excessive sun exposure. Use long-sleeved clothing and sunscreen to shield your at-risk arm from sunburn, which can exacerbate lymphoedema. Your skin's integrity is paramount.

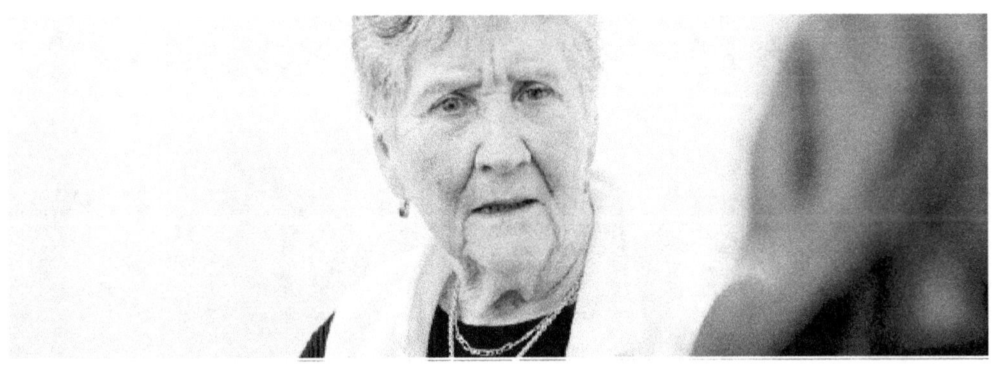

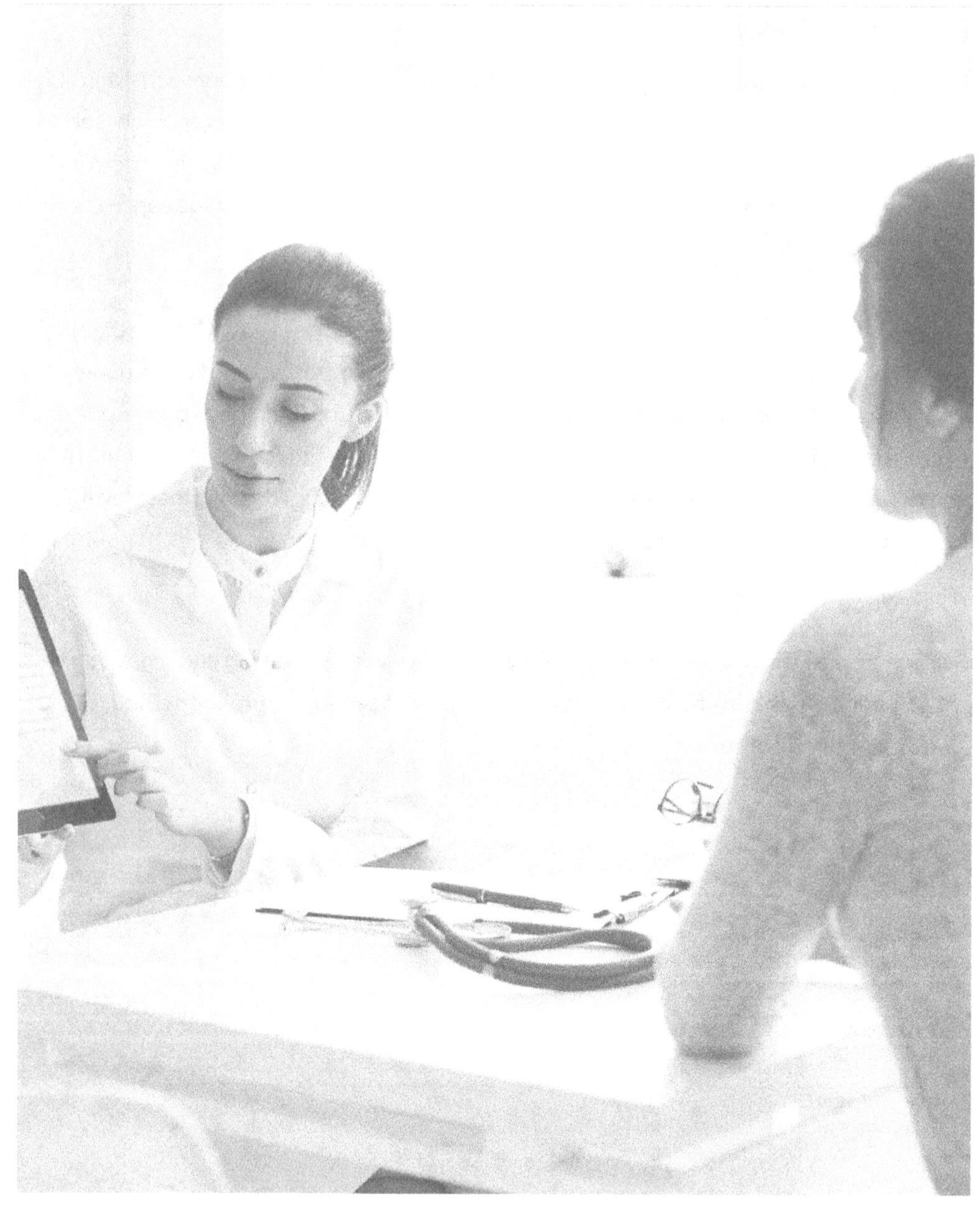

3.4 Can Needles Trigger Lymphoedema?

I want to delve into a crucial topic: the potential link between needle injections and the onset of lymphoedema.

Firstly, let's understand why we emphasize avoiding needlestick penetration on the affected arm, which refers to the arm where lymph nodes have been removed due to breast cancer treatment. It's essential to note that this might apply to one or both arms, depending on your treatment history, as having lymph nodes removed from one or both armpits or undergoing radiation therapy can put you at risk of developing lymphoedema.

The guidelines typically advise patients to avoid needlestick procedures on the affected arm. Specifically, we're talking about three common types of needlestick procedures: vaccinations, infusions, and blood draw.

It's crucial to recognize that the real issue isn't the initial needle penetration itself but the complications that can arise from it. For instance, if a healthcare provider struggles to find a vein, leading to multiple attempts and subsequent inflammation and bruising around the injection site, this can potentially trigger lymphoedema.

Let's break down these needlestick procedures:

Vaccinations: Vaccinations introduce inactive viruses into your arm, inducing an immune response. Since lymph nodes are part of your immune system, vaccinations can overtax your lymphatic system if you've had lymph nodes removed from your affected arm. Therefore, it's wise to opt for the non-affected side when getting vaccinated.

Blood Pressure Testing: While I've never personally witnessed lymphoedema triggered immediately after a blood pressure test, there have been documented cases. Thus, using the unaffected arm for blood pressure readings is recommended when possible.

If you've had lymph nodes removed, radiation therapy, or are otherwise at risk of lymphoedema, the overarching message is clear: opt for the arm without lymph node involvement whenever possible for vaccinations, infusions, blood draws, and blood pressure tests.

So, what can you do to ensure your voice is heard when a healthcare provider attempts a procedure on your affected arm? First and foremost, educate yourself on the potential risks and share this knowledge with friends, family, and colleagues who are at risk of lymphoedema. Knowledge is power, and spreading awareness can make a significant difference.

Consider using a medical alert band that clearly states your situation, such as "No blood pressure tests" and "No needles on this arm." These bands can be instrumental if undergoing multiple procedures or hospitalizations.

Lastly, don't hesitate to communicate your needs with your medical team. Whether you're scheduled for surgery, sedation, or any medical procedure, ensure that the healthcare providers understand the importance of avoiding needlestick penetration on your affected arm.

As noted earlier in this chapter, provide verbal communication and documentation to alert your Medical Team regarding your lack of consent to using the affected arm.

If you know you will have difficulty standing up to a Medical Professional who is putting pressure on you to be able to use the affected arm, consider taking a support person or advocate with you to the appointment. While the research around risk of needlestick penetration and lymphoedema may not be gold standard, there are certainly a number of cases I can attest to over the last decade where needle stick injury has created potential cases of lymphoedema.

Whether you're at risk of lymphoedema or already have it, the consensus remains: avoid vaccinations, infusions, blood draws, and blood pressure tests on the affected arm. Your commitment to these precautions can significantly impact your overall health and well-being.

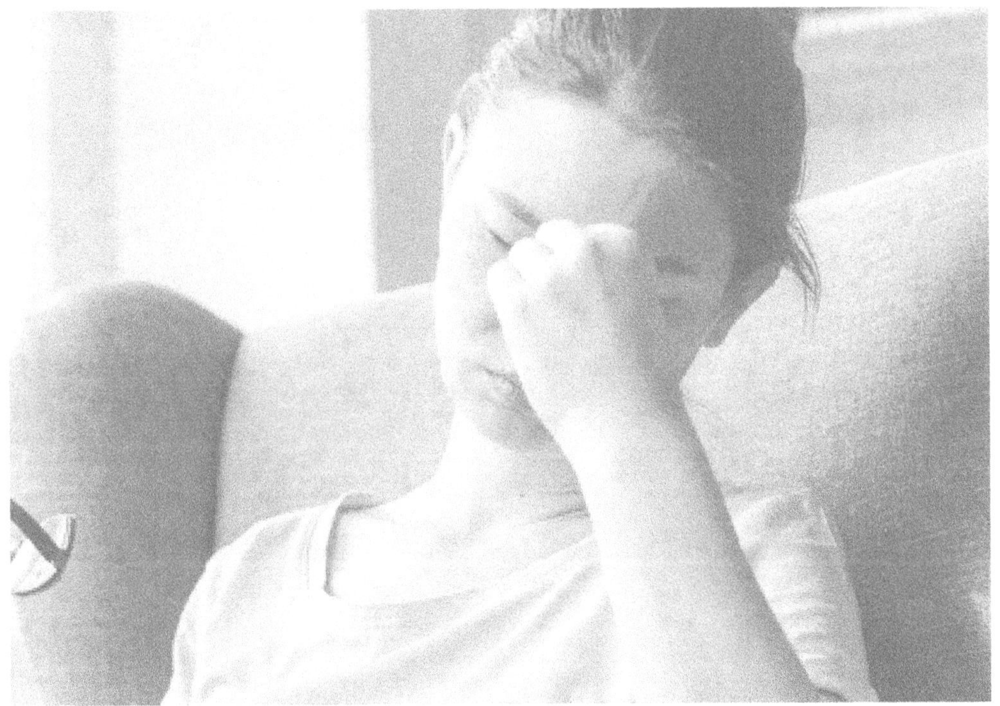

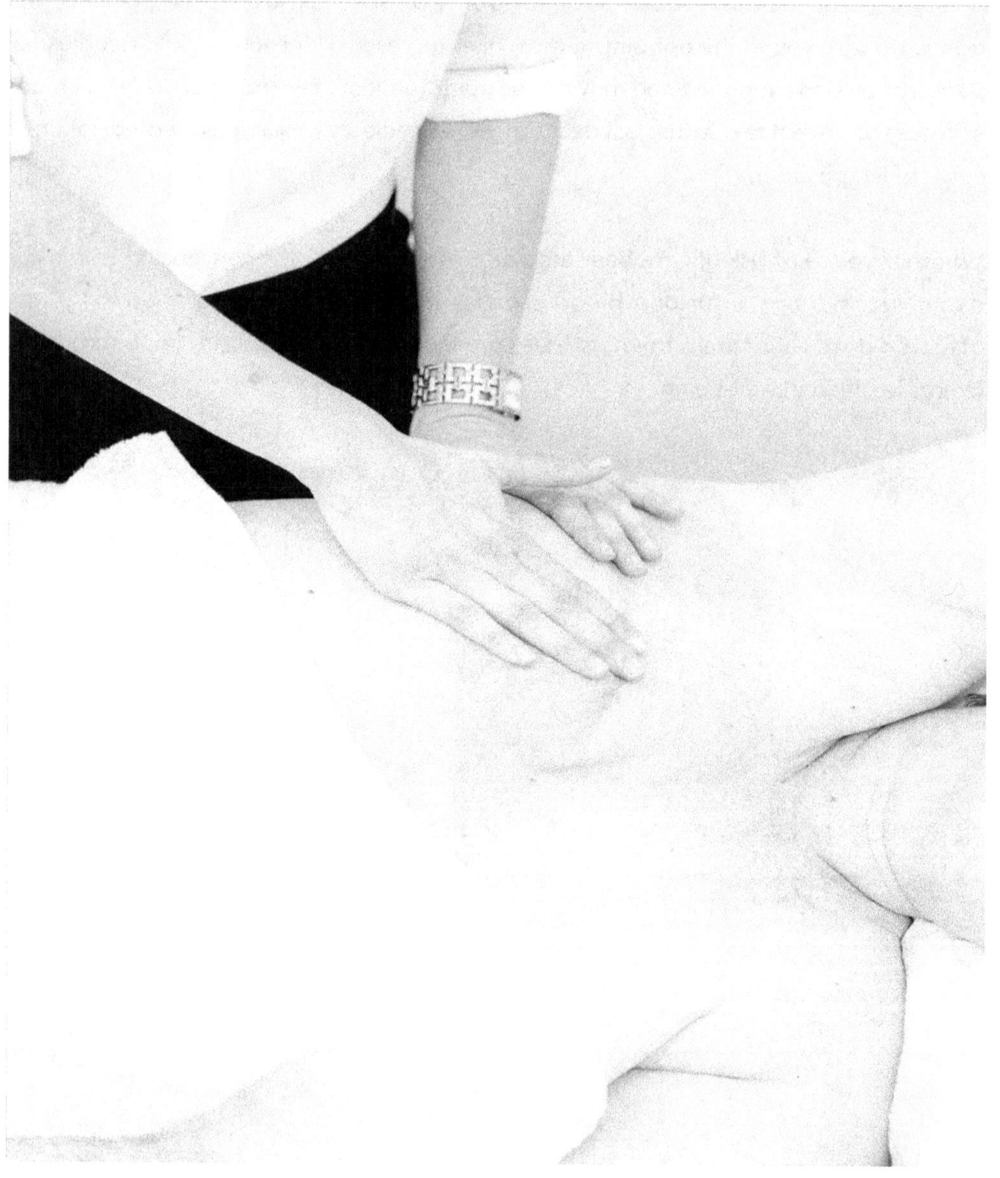

3.5 Self-Lymphatic Drainage Massage for Breast Cancer Patients

This section will explore the importance of performing self-lymphatic drainage massage. This technique can be really valuable if you deal with existing or early-onset lymphoedema following breast cancer treatment.

First, let's establish what self-lymphatic drainage massage entails. This technique involves clearing excess lymphatic fluid in the upper limb or breast. It can be done independently (self-lymphatic drainage) or with the assistance of another person (manual lymphatic drainage). In this context, we'll focus on self-lymphatic drainage.

The technique of self-lymphatic drainage massage has evolved, with a significant breakthrough in 2019 by researchers at Macquarie University in Sydney, Australia. Traditionally, this massage employed feather-light pressure and aimed to redirect fluid from the affected arm, to the opposite armpit or towards the groin, where other lymph node fields are located. The original assumption made was that if a woman had undergone an axillary lymph node dissection (i.e. all lymph nodes removed from an armpit), that this armpit would not be able to take up any excess lymphatic fluid that was drained to it by manual (or self) lymphatic drainage.

However, recent research has revealed a more practical approach. Regardless of the number of lymph nodes removed during treatment, it has been found that draining fluid to the same armpit on the same side as the affected limb is the most efficient method (Koelmeyer et al, 2020). This groundbreaking discovery shifts our perspective on how to manage lymphoedema effectively.

The other major finding from the same study involved a significant change in the pressures used during lymphatic drainage massage. The research found that firm (but not painful) pressure was more effective than feather-light pressure. I often tell my patients who are prescribed Self Lymphatic Drainage, to think of their arm like a sponge full of water: slow, firm pressure squeezed on the sponge will be the most effective pressure to get all of the water drained out. Light pressure on the sponge will get a few drops out, but won't be anywhere near as effective as slow, firm pressure.

So, let's explore how to perform self-lymphatic drainage massage:

Step 1: Stimulate Your Lymph Node Field

Raise your arm and use your four fingers to perform a firm, circular massage in your armpit. This massage stimulates your lymph node field, even if you've had all lymph nodes removed. You can repeat this process in the small area just above your collarbone.

Step 2: Clear the Upper Arm

Begin clearing the upper arm section, treating the arm like a cylinder. Apply firm (but not painful) pressure, ensuring you massage all areas, including the arm's front, back, and underside. Always direct the fluid toward the same armpit on the affected side.

Step 3: Clear the Hand and Forearm

Start with the back of your hand, working through the forearm, and include the spaces between your fingers. Note: if you can't see or feel any excess fluid in your fingers and hand, you can focus your massage on the forearm. Use firm pressure to move the lymphatic fluid up the forearm and the entire arm's length, maintaining the same direction towards the affected armpit.

Step 4: Re-stimulate Your Lymph Node Field

Repeat the circular, firm massage in your armpit and the area above the collarbone for 10 to 20 seconds.

Now, let's address some common questions and practical considerations:

Frequency and Duration: The frequency and duration of self-lymphatic drainage massage depends on individual circumstances and practicality. Research suggests that 30 to 45 minutes of massage tends to plateau lymphatic fluid movement. However, shorter sessions performed frequently may be more manageable for many. Early-stage lymphoedema may require shorter, more frequent sessions, while severe cases could benefit from longer sessions. The key is regularity but also consider your own circumstances. Some massage is better than none, but make sure you are performing massage in a manner that is sustainable for you.

Prevention of Lymphoedema: At the time of writing this book, research suggests that self-lymphatic drainage massage does not necessarily prevent lymphoedema but can be a valuable tool in managing it. Hence I rarely encourage women who are only at risk of lymphoedema to perform regular self lymphatic drainage. This is a surprise to many women who do not have lymphoedema, but if there is no excess fluid on their affected arm, it should suggest that their lymphatic system is performing capably and does not necessarily require extra assistance.

Self Lymphatic Drainage is just one component of a comprehensive approach that includes compression garments, exercise, limb elevation, and skincare.

When Not to Perform Self-Lymphatic Drainage: Avoid self-lymphatic drainage massage if you have an active infection anywhere in your body, not just the affected limb. Seek medical advice before resuming the massage in such cases.

Additional Tips: Deep breathing enhances lymphatic flow, so incorporate it into your massage routine. Elevating your arm while massaging further aids fluid drainage. If you experience discomfort holding your arm up, support your shoulder with a stable object nearby. Use a non-irritating moisturizer or cream to prevent skin drag during the massage. Consider performing the massage before bedtime to avoid the challenge of putting on a compression garment over moisturized skin. Finally, establish a consistent time or activity during the day for your self-lymphatic drainage routine to ensure it becomes a regular habit.

Self-lymphatic drainage massage is a valuable self-care practice for breast cancer patients with lymphoedema. By integrating it into your daily routine, you can take proactive steps toward managing this condition and enhancing your overall well-being. Remember that consistency is key on this journey to improved health and vitality.

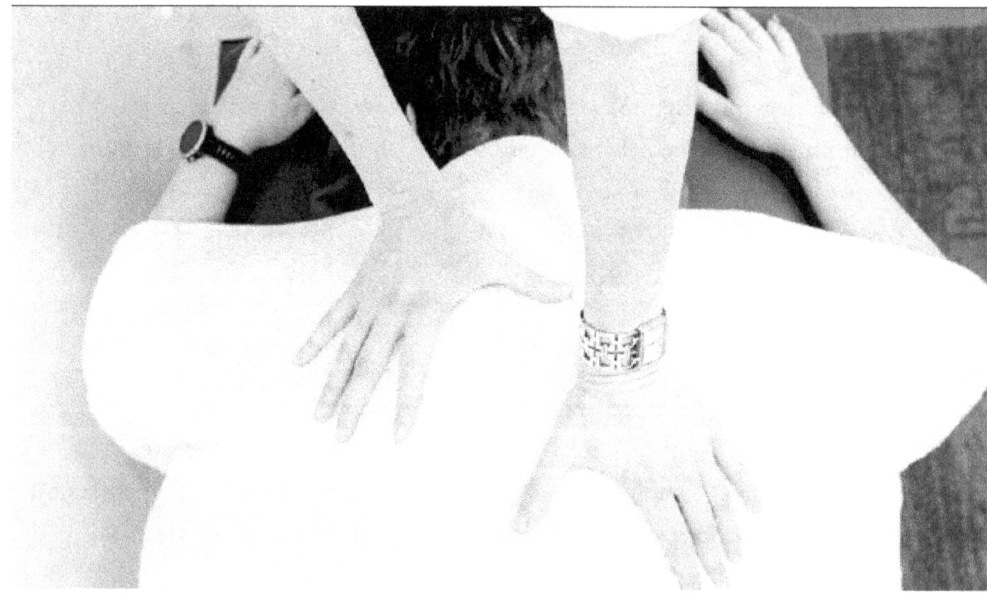

3.6 Lymphatic Drainage for Breast Swelling: A Comprehensive Guide

In this topic, I will guide you through lymphatic drainage massage techniques tailored explicitly for breast swelling.

Let's dive right into the topic by addressing some crucial points before delving into the massage technique.

Understanding Breast Swelling: When Does it Occur? Breast tissue swelling can manifest at various stages during or after breast cancer treatment. The two most common scenarios are:

Postoperative Edema: After breast surgery, such as a lumpectomy, some individuals may experience postoperative swelling or edema. This is a natural side effect of surgery and should not be immediately classified as lymphoedema. Recognizing that acute swelling can often be treated effectively if addressed promptly is crucial.

Swelling After Radiation: Breast swelling can occur during or after radiation therapy. Just like postoperative edema, this type of swelling may not necessarily indicate lymphoedema. Identifying it correctly and taking timely action is essential.

I want to emphasize that not all breast swelling is lymphoedema, especially when it initially appears. Jumping to conclusions can be counterproductive. Rather than immediately labelling it as lymphoedema, consider it edema, allowing for a more pragmatic approach to treatment.

When to Seek Medical Attention: It's prudent to consult your medical team if you experience side effects of treatment, there are several reasons to seek medical advice:

- Ensuring the type of swelling and its cause is correctly identified.
- Rule out complications such as seromas or hematomas.
- Address possible infections, which may exhibit signs like redness, fever, and increased discomfort.

Seeking professional guidance in these situations helps ensure the appropriate course of action.

Let's explore how to perform lymphatic drainage for breast swelling based on the most recent studies and clinical experience.

Direction of Lymphatic Drainage: The drainage pathways in breast tissue changes once one or more lymph nodes have been removed during breast cancer surgery (Heydon-White, 2020). In such cases, it's important to note the following:

- You can typically drain the breast towards the same-side armpit for individuals without lymph node removal on the affected side.
- However, if one or more lymph nodes have been removed, the drainage pathway often shifts towards the breastbone (sternum), the collarbone (clavicle), or even the opposite armpit.

Keep these pathways in mind while performing the massage. Considering the large majority of women require at least one lymph node to be removed during Breast Cancer surgery, most women will need to perform lymphatic drainage on their breast in a direction that is towards the breastbone and or collarbone.

Pressure: When it comes to the pressure applied during the massage, research suggests that slow, firm pressure is more effective for lymphatic drainage massage. While light pressure is safe, clinical experience indicates that slow, firm pressure can yield better results.

Frequency: The frequency of breast lymphatic drainage massage is an important consideration. To avoid overexertion and soreness, it's recommended to perform the massage once a day, ideally for 5 to 10 minutes. Consistency is key. Frequent, shorter sessions are more beneficial than infrequent, extended ones. Some of my patients have tried to be too diligent and have ended up with a sore breast because they have performed massages multiple times every day of the week.

Now, let's discuss the massage technique itself:

1. Choose a Comfortable Hand: Start using the hand that feels most comfortable. If you're dealing with swelling in the left breast, using the right hand is common, and vice versa.

2. Position Yourself: For self-massage, find a comfortable position and keep your arm out of the way. You can place your hand on your head or shoulder to achieve this.

Note: I often suggest to my patients that performing this massage in the shower is a common sense time hack as you are already undressed and hopefully warm and comfortable. I recommend leaving a bottle of moisturiser in the shower so that this becomes a daily ritual that you don't have to make spare time for.

3. Massage Technique: Begin by applying slow, firm pressure to push fluid from the breast base towards either the breastbone (sternum) or the collarbone (clavicle), depending on the direction indicated by your treatment history. This massage movement helps facilitate lymphatic drainage.

Remember, performing lymphatic drainage massage on yourself might not be as effective as when done by a therapist. However, it is a valuable self-care practice that can reduce breast swelling and improve your comfort. It is also an opportunity to work on tight scar tissue from your Breast surgery.

In conclusion, this comprehensive guide aims to empower you with the knowledge and techniques needed to address breast swelling, whether you're a healthcare practitioner, a breast cancer survivor, or a patient. Following these guidelines, you can take proactive steps to manage and alleviate breast swelling, promoting your overall well-being and quality of life.

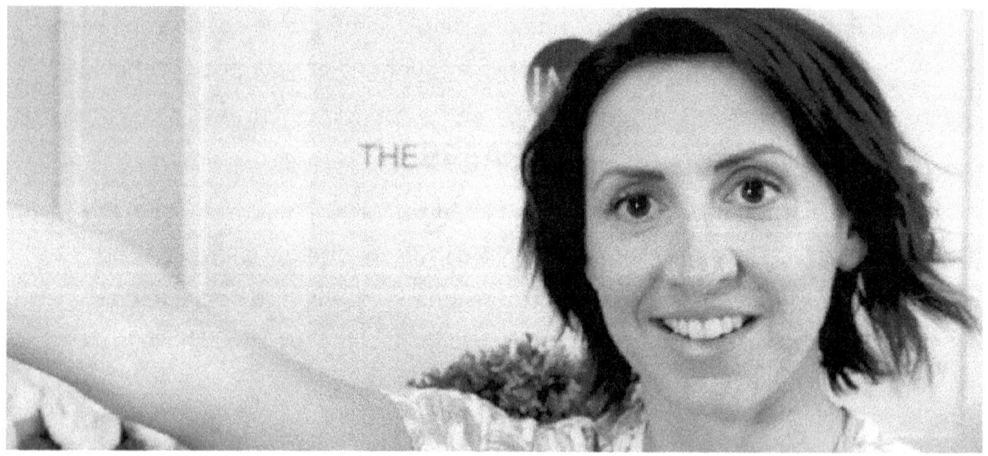

BREAST CANCER REVOLUTION

Jen McKenzie

Remember to access your goodies in the
BCR Resource Vault.
Scan the QR code above to Access.

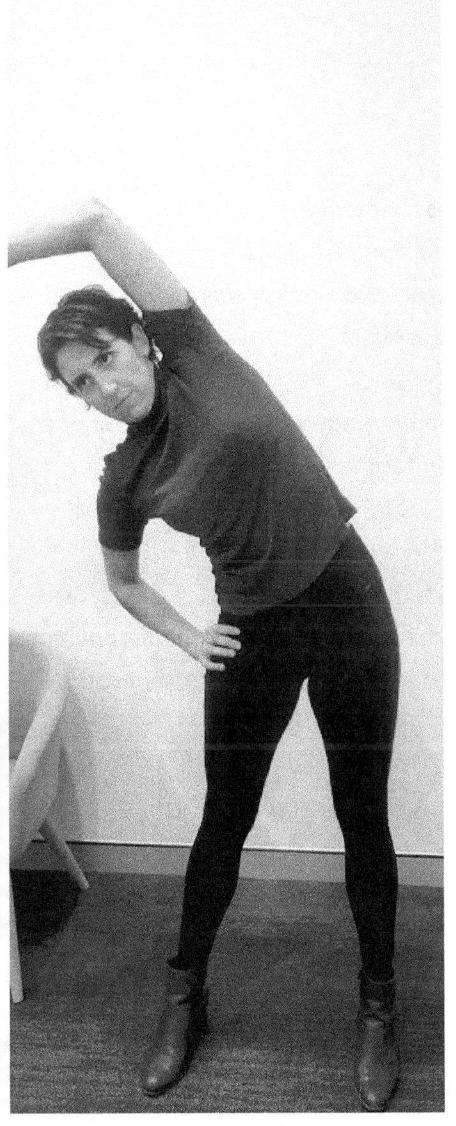

Empowering Movement:

Harnessing the Benefits of Exercise and Lymphatic Drainage in Breast Cancer Recovery

4.1 Unlocking the Benefits of Exercise During and After Breast Cancer

My focus in this chapter centres on the top six reasons why exercise is vital to managing breast cancer during and after treatment, for both Breast Cancer survivors, and Breast Cancer patients.

1. Combat the Side Effects of Breast Cancer Treatment

Breast cancer treatment often ushers in a wave of challenging side effects. These can be physically and emotionally taxing, leaving patients searching for effective coping methods. Exercise emerges as a powerful ally in this battle.

Consider the fatigue that frequently accompanies chemotherapy and radiation. While the instinct may be to rest and conserve energy, current research strongly suggests that exercise can counteract fatigue effectively (Cormie et al, 2018). It might seem counterintuitive, but physical activity can help manage this common side effect.

Similarly, exercise can be an antidote to chemotherapy-induced nausea, providing relief when needed. Moreover, weight gain is a concern for many during breast cancer treatment, but regular exercise can help maintain body weight, keeping it within a healthy range.

Fluid retention, often exacerbated by steroids administered during chemotherapy, can also be mitigated through exercise. By promoting regular fluid flushing, exercise assists in alleviating this common discomfort.

2. Improve Muscle Mass

Breast cancer treatment can lead to a decline in muscle mass and strength, a condition known as deconditioning. In particular, chemotherapy alone accelerates muscle mass loss. This reduction in muscle mass, otherwise known as muscle atrophy, can make even simple tasks, like lifting objects or walking up a set of stairs, arduous.

Furthermore, individuals who have completed their breast cancer treatment might still grapple with the physical repercussions of insufficient post-treatment rehabilitation. Exercise is a key solution for addressing muscle mass loss and regaining strength.

It's crucial to note that appearances can be deceiving. Some individuals may appear slim but lack essential muscle mass. Consider a body composition analysis test to understand your body composition better. This test can reveal the proportion of fatty tissue, muscle, and fluid in your body, shedding light on whether you need to focus on rebuilding muscle for energy and strength.

3. Lessen the Risk of Osteoporosis

Breast cancer treatment including chemotherapy and certain hormone blockers, as well as menopause, can collectively increase the risk of low bone mineral density, also known as osteoporosis. Osteopenia, a precursor to osteoporosis, is another concern.

Chemotherapy, in particular, doubles the risk of developing low bone mineral density compared to that of the general population (Boehnke Michaud & Goodin, 2006). Additionally, post-menopausal women, who constitute a significant portion of breast cancer patients, face reduced oestrogen levels, further impacting bone health. Hormone-blocking medications, namely Aromatase Inhibitors, prescribed to oestrogen-positive breast cancer patients can also significantly reduce bone mineral density.

The solution lies in resistance exercise (or lifting weights) and weight-bearing activities like walking. These forms of exercise effectively combat the decline in bone mineral density, offering a proactive approach to preserving bone health. Other treatment options are available, such as bone stock injections and infusions, but when it comes to exercise, the gold standard for improving bone mineral density is resistance training.

4. Improve Mental Health

Breast cancer brings a cascade of emotional challenges, often leaving individuals grappling with fear, stress, anxiety, depression, anger, and overwhelm. Mental health support during and after breast cancer is essential yet frequently underemphasized.

Exercise is something that you can be in complete control of during and following your diagnosis, and this in itself is empowering. It can feel as if so many things in your life have been taken out of your control. But this is where the tool that is exercise is different: You can choose where to exercise, how you will exercise, who you will exercise with, what environment you exercise in and how many times a week you will perform exercise.

Exercise can be a powerful tool for enhancing mental well-being. It triggers the release of endorphins, our natural "feel-good" hormones. This surge of positivity can make a significant difference in your overall outlook and emotional resilience.

Moreover, exercise provides a break from the clinical settings commonly associated with cancer treatment. It offers a chance to step outside, breathe fresh air, and connect with the world beyond hospital walls or medical centres. Even engaging in a supportive exercise community, whether at a gym or in group classes, can help individuals feel less isolated.

Exercise also plays a role in reducing brain fog (previously referred to as 'chemo brain'). Regular physical activity reduces stress and inflammation, and improves cerebral blood flow (blood flow to the brain), all of which can help to reduce cognitive difficulties often experienced during and following treatment (Downs et al, 2023).

5. Improve Energy Levels

Fighting fatigue is a common concern for individuals undergoing breast cancer treatment. Fatigue can be debilitating, affecting one's daily life and sense of normalcy. However, exercise provides a powerful means to combat this exhaustion.

It's essential to clarify that exercise doesn't demand marathon-level exertion. Starting slowly and gently is perfectly acceptable, especially when you're fatigued and trying to work out what your body will cope with at different phases of your treatment or recovery. Gentle activities such as yoga, aqua aerobics, or a leisurely walk can be a starting point. The goal is not to exhaust yourself but to gradually build energy levels. I often say to my patients: I don't care where you start, I care where you finish.

The research stresses the significance of avoiding a sedentary lifestyle during breast cancer treatment. Regular, moderate-intensity exercise sessions-2-3 times a week-can significantly reduce fatigue and enhance overall well-being, not to mention reduce your risk of Breast Cancer recurring.

6. Lymphoedema Prevention

Lymphoedema is a potential side effect of breast cancer treatment characterized by chronic swelling in the arm, particularly when lymph nodes have been removed. Prevention and management are key concerns for breast cancer patients.

Engaging in regular resistance training, even a couple of times a week at a moderate intensity, has shown a remarkable reduction in the risk of lymphoedema development by over 70%. This statistic is based on a comprehensive study conducted a decade ago. Despite the age of the study, it was very well performed research on a large number of Breast Cancer patients and I certainly see evidence of the paper's findings today (Schmitz et al, 2009).

Additionally, this research also found that regular resistance exercise can reduce the likelihood of lymphoedema flare-ups by more than 50% for those already managing lymphoedema. It's a proactive approach to safeguarding your well-being.

In summary, exercise during and after breast cancer treatment is beneficial and often essential. It helps manage treatment side effects, maintains muscle mass and strength, and reduces the risk of osteoporosis. Exercise is a multifaceted ally in the breast cancer journey, improving mental health, boosting energy levels, and significantly reducing the risk of lymphoedema. These benefits, combined with exercise's potential to diminish the risk of breast cancer recurrence, underscore its vital role in the lives of breast cancer survivors and patients. Embrace exercise as a source of empowerment and healing on your path to recovery.

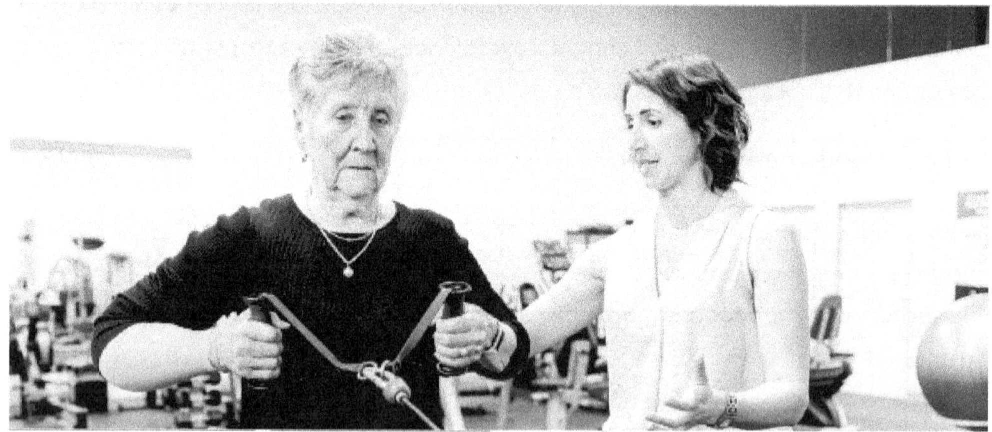

4.2 Rediscovering the Joy of Exercise After Breast Cancer Treatment

In this chapter, I want to tackle a challenge that many breast cancer survivors face once treatment concludes: how to regain motivation for exercise. Emerging from the strenuous journey of breast cancer treatment, it's common to feel lost in terms of returning to your usual physical activity or exercise. I'm here to guide you through this transitional phase, offering insights and strategies to help you rekindle your motivation and start exercising again.

Understanding the Motivation Dilemma

Surviving breast cancer is a remarkable achievement, and the focus during treatment is understandably on survival. However, this period often takes a toll on your overall well-being. Nutritional habits may suffer, exercise routines may be neglected, and a sense of fatigue sets in. When treatment ends, the prospect of returning to exercise can be daunting, even though you recognize its importance.

It's crucial to understand that the lack of motivation to exercise is a remarkably common issue, and you are not alone in experiencing it. In this chapter, I'll share six valuable tips to help you overcome this mental hurdle and re-establish a fulfilling exercise routine.

Tip 1: Set the Psychological Bar Low

The first and perhaps most important tip is to set the bar as low as possible regarding your initial exercise expectations. Many individuals envision an intense workout regimen akin to running a marathon when they think about resuming exercise. This can be overwhelming and deter you from even starting. Or worse, you start an exercise routine that IS overwhelming and stop after only a few sessions because it is too much for you mentally and maybe even physically.

Instead, start with the smallest, simplest form of exercise possible. For example, your first session could consist of a leisurely walk around your neighbourhood or 10 minutes of gentle yoga in the comfort of your home. Keeping your initial goals attainable makes it easier to overcome the mental barrier and build momentum. If your first few sessions feel too easy, no problem-use it as an indication that you are ready to progress onto something a little more challenging.

Tip 2: Begin Without Breaking a Sweat

Avoid the misconception that exercise must be gruelling, sweaty, and physically demanding (although later on you are certainly welcome to return to it looking and feeling like this!). When you're in the early stages of resuming exercise, focus on gentle activities that don't make you break a sweat. This could include activities like basic yoga sessions or walking at a comfortable pace. The objective is to reintroduce your body to movement without overwhelming yourself physically or mentally.

Tip 3: Don't Overdo It

At the start, limit your exercise frequency to a couple of weekly sessions. Going from zero to hero, attempting to complete intense workouts daily, is not sustainable and may lead to burnout or excessive soreness. Gradually ease into your exercise routine. As your body adapts, you can increase your workout frequency and intensity.

Breast Cancer treatment often involves chemotherapy which can significantly impact aerobic capacity. Overwhelm can occur quickly if you push beyond your aerobic limits when first getting started. This can be stressful and upsetting for many women who are trying to do the right thing by getting back into exercise but have put too much pressure on themselves at the start.

Remember, the goal isn't to push yourself to the limit immediately but to create a sustainable exercise habit you can build upon over time. Allow yourself the grace to progress gradually. By all means, you are absolutely welcome and encouraged to aim for a return to competitive sport or high-intensity exercise if this is your goal but remember where you are starting from and what your mind and body have just gone through.

Tip 4: Small Progressions Are Key

As you reacquaint yourself with exercise, making small progressions in intensity, frequency, and duration is vital. Avoid jumping from one level to another in pursuit of rapid results. Gradual, manageable progressions will prevent muscle soreness and reduce the risk of lymphoedema.

For instance, if you've started with a simple resistance training program, aim to increase your weights by just one or two kilograms at a time. If walking is your chosen form of exercise, consider extending your walking route by a small distance rather than attempting a significant leap in distance. Small steps toward progression will help you achieve your goals while minimizing the risk of setbacks.

Tip 5: Just Put Your Shoes On

One of the greatest adversaries to exercise motivation is the stream of excuses that your mind conjures. Overcoming this mental hurdle can be as simple as putting on your exercise shoes. When your brain begins to list why you shouldn't exercise, ignore it.

Instead, focus on this singular task: putting on your exercise shoes.

Once your shoes are on, you'll often find that you've overcome the mental barriers holding you back. This small action can be the catalyst for a successful exercise session. Walking is a fantastic, equipment-free way to initiate this habit. You only need comfortable shoes and a safe place to walk.

Keep it simple, and let putting on your shoes become your gateway to regular exercise. Women are fantastic at overthinking things - sometimes it is best to "do" rather than "think".

Tip 6: Set Yourself a Short-Term Goal

Having a clear goal with a specific time frame can be a powerful motivator. Whether signing up for a charity run, committing to walk a certain distance with a friend, or reaching a fitness milestone, setting short-term goals helps keep you accountable and provides a sense of purpose.

Your goals should be realistic and tailored to your current fitness level. Don't shy away from setting the bar low if it means achieving it is within reach. The sense of accomplishment from achieving these goals will boost your confidence and motivation, putting you on the path to long-term success.

Remember, the journey to reignite your exercise motivation is unique to you. It's about simplifying the process and finding what works best for your situation. Following these tips and focusing on gradual progress, you can overcome the motivation slump and embark on your exercise journey with renewed enthusiasm.

BREAST
CANCER
REVOLUTION

Jen McKenzie

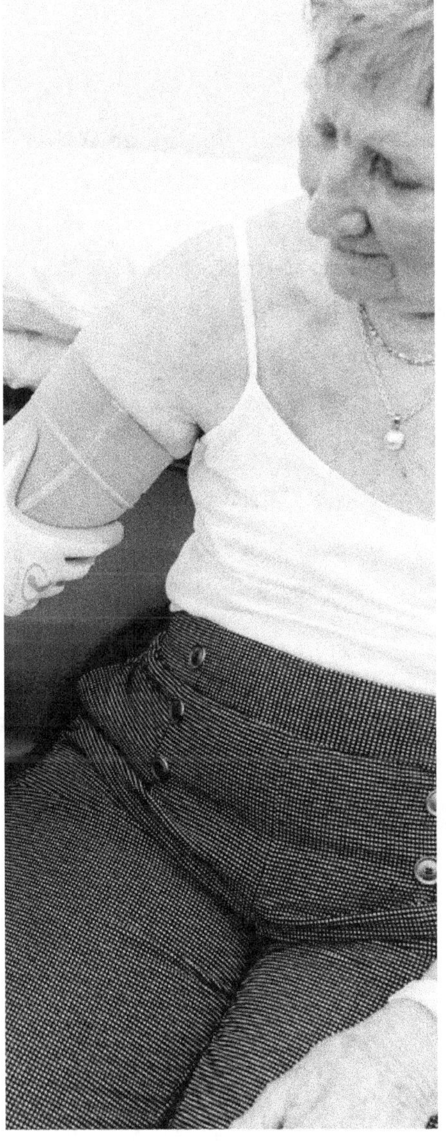

Restoring Movement:

Unlocking Shoulder Mobility in Breast Cancer Recovery

In this important chapter, we aim to shed light on a crucial aspect that demands the attention of healthcare practitioners, breast cancer survivors, and patients alike: the significance of restoring shoulder range of motion following breast cancer surgery. Our mission is to impart essential knowledge about why this endeavour deserves significant attention following Breast Cancer surgery.

We will elucidate the top six compelling reasons why regaining shoulder mobility should be a primary focus in your post-surgery journey.

1. Shoulder Mobility and Its Importance in Daily Life.

For those transitioning directly from surgery to radiation, irrespective of whether they underwent a lumpectomy or mastectomy, the demand for a significantly elevated shoulder position during radiation sessions underscores the vital importance of restoring mobility to this joint. The implications of failing to do so, including the potential development of cording, tight scar tissue, or persistent shoulder discomfort, are topics we will explore in detail.

In this journey, your physiotherapist is central to your support team, who plays a pivotal role in helping you regain shoulder mobility through various exercises and manual therapies, such as massage and joint mobilization. Physiotherapists will highlight the importance of how your treatment regimen and its sequence can impact your shoulder mobility, particularly when radiation therapy immediately follows surgery.

Furthermore, we will elucidate the challenges posed by a moderately stiff shoulder when entering radiation therapy, which often spans three to six weeks with daily appointments. Patients frequently find themselves in an elevated position for up to 15 minutes during these sessions. Failure to maintain adequate shoulder mobility can result in worsening stiffness and discomfort as radiation progresses, potentially increasing the risk of shoulder bursitis, a topic we will explore further.

Early Physiotherapy that continues during the early weeks of radiation can be vital for many patients to complete their radiation treatment without worsening shoulder symptoms.

2. Ability to Engage in Essential Functional Activities.

It may appear inconspicuous, but the significance of a mobile shoulder becomes profoundly evident when we consider the myriad of ways our daily lives rely on this body part. This realization often dawns upon us only when an injury or restriction occurs.

This encompassing functionality extends across diverse aspects of life, from pursuing athletic endeavours like sports or yoga, where a stiff or restricted shoulder can significantly impede one's performance. Household chores, a quintessential part of daily living, can also be dramatically impacted by poor shoulder mobility.

Tasks as basic as cleaning a window or reaching for items on an overhead shelf demand a healthy range of motion in your shoulder to be performed with ease.

Moreover, we confront scenarios where restricted shoulder mobility curtails our participation in activities we hold dear, particularly during holidays. The inability to partake in a game of tennis or enjoy the simple pleasure of swimming due to shoulder limitations underscores the far-reaching impact of shoulder mobility on our quality of life.

3. To Prevent Lymphoedema.

To comprehend the link between shoulder mobility and lymphoedema, it is crucial to delve into the physiology of the lymphatic system. Unlike the arterial system, which benefits from the forceful pumping action of the heart and can thus expel blood with vigour if an artery is cut, the lymphatic system operates differently.

Without a major central pump, it relies heavily on muscle contractions, gravity and movement to facilitate the movement of lymphatic fluid.

Herein lies the crux: a stiff or immobile shoulder can inadvertently impede the muscle contractions necessary for lymph fluid circulation. When assessing strategies for lymphoedema prevention, it becomes imperative to consider an individual's capacity to move their shoulder. The rigidity of the shoulder joint can reduce the flow of lymphatic fluid, potentially increasing risk of developing lymphoedema.

Furthermore, elevating the affected arm is one of the recommended therapeutic approaches for those who have already developed lymphoedema. This elevation capitalizes on gravity's assistance to encourage lymphatic fluid to drain back down the arm. However, if your shoulder mobility is severely restricted, achieving the necessary arm elevation becomes a formidable challenge, limiting the effectiveness of this treatment strategy.

4. To Regain Full Strength.

Imagine being able to perform tasks below shoulder height effortlessly but struggling with movements that require lifting your arm overhead due to factors such as scar tissue or musculoskeletal tension. This limitation means that a significant portion of your shoulder remains weak. Weakness tends to create tension, and the interplay between weakness and tension often results in pain. Therefore, one of the most compelling motivations to reestablish shoulder range of motion after breast cancer surgery is to regain the ability to perform everyday activities with a normal, pain-free shoulder. Whether performing a lat pull-down at the gym, pushing against a resistance band, or lifting a dumbbell, having a functional shoulder is crucial for maintaining an active lifestyle. This holds true even for individuals who may not consider themselves regular gym-goers, as restricted shoulder mobility can unexpectedly affect daily life.

5. Pain Relief

As mentioned, limited range of motion often increases tissue tension and persistent weakness. This cycle eventually culminates in one inevitable outcome: pain. After breast cancer surgery, it's not uncommon to experience discomfort and tightness in the shoulder region, with the back of the shoulder blade being a frequent trouble spot. While there are techniques like using a tennis ball for self-massage to alleviate this discomfort, seeking the expertise of a physiotherapist experienced in treating breast cancer patients or even a massage therapist knowledgeable about the necessary precautions for post-surgical care can be immensely beneficial. Sometimes the number of treatment sessions required to 'free up' an area of tight tissue can be surprisingly small, but the benefits can be amazing.

This is a critical point to discuss because following breast cancer surgery, the accumulation of muscular tension, especially in the shoulder area, is prevalent. This tension can manifest behind the shoulder blade and in muscles like the pectoralis and upper trapezius. Ultimately, this tension can lead to both restricted shoulder mobility, weakness and in turn, pain. Therefore, alleviating pain is paramount in enhancing the quality of life for breast cancer survivors, and addressing shoulder mobility plays a vital role in achieving this goal.

6. Reduce the Risk of Cording

Despite cording not yet being defined medically, from my clinical experience cording is extreme nerve tension. Cording represents nerve tension that typically arises following axillary lymph node dissection or sentinel node biopsy. Whenever surgical procedures are performed in the axillary region, there's a general susceptibility to developing cording, and an important correlation emerges-the stiffer the shoulder's range of motion, the more difficult it is to treat and resolve cording.

However, a key insight is that superior shoulder range of motion considerably eases the treatment of cording. Therefore, it's imperative to remember that our goal extends beyond averting lymphoedema; we're also actively working to minimize the risk of cording when we prioritize restoring shoulder range of motion in breast cancer recovery.

We've set out on a journey in this chapter to discover the many-faceted causes behind the critical requirement to regain shoulder mobility following breast cancer surgery. The shoulder's importance in the post-surgery recovery process cannot be overstated, as it aids in daily activities, prevents lymphoedema, aids in strength recovery, reduces pain, and allows for faster treatment and resolution of cording.

As you reflect on my comprehensive insights, remember that this knowledge is a powerful tool in your breast cancer recovery arsenal. Empowered with this understanding, you can make informed decisions and collaborate effectively with your healthcare team to ensure that shoulder mobility is not overlooked on your path to a healthier, more vibrant life beyond breast cancer.

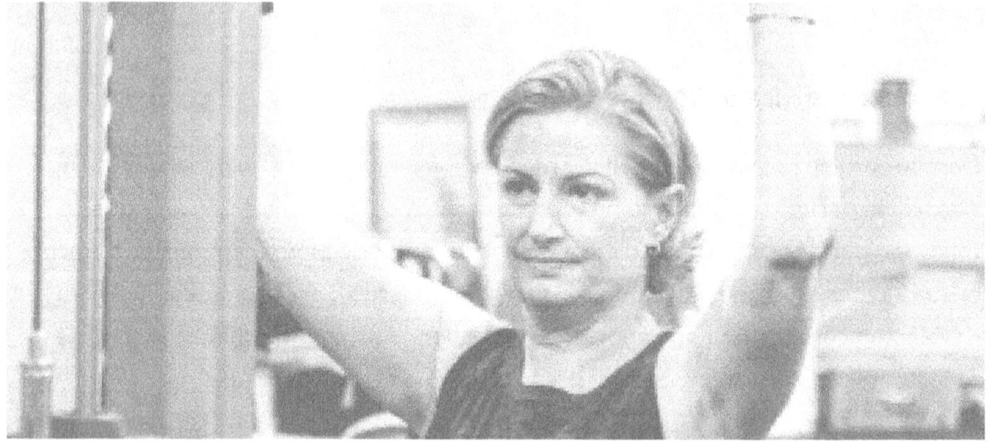

BREAST CANCER REVOLUTION

Jen McKenzie

Remember to access your goodies in the
BCR Resource Vault.
Scan the QR code above to Access.

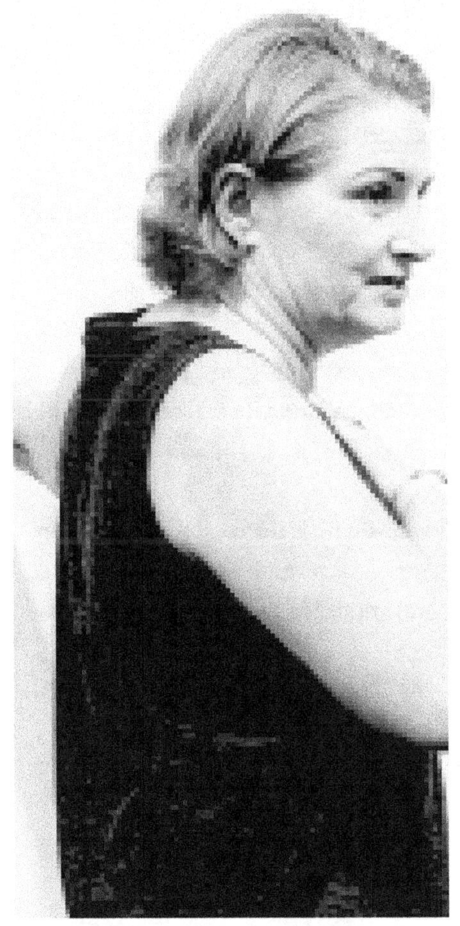

Restoring Inner Radiance:

Overcoming the Mental
Challenges of Breast
Cancer Recovery

6.1 Navigating Emotional Well-being During and After Breast Cancer: The Unspoken Struggle

In this chapter, I'm shifting the focus from the physical aspects of breast cancer to a topic that affects countless women following diagnosis: their emotional well-being during and after the journey. It's a theme that has resonated with many of my patients, and I felt compelled to address it because it often remains unspoken. So, let's delve into the heart of the matter: that moment when you're walking down the street, whether you're in the midst of breast cancer treatment or on the road to recovery, and someone, be it a family member, friend, coworker, or neighbour, says those familiar words, "Oh wow, you look great." And while you reply with a polite, "Thanks, I feel great".

But secretly you think, "I don't feel great. I feel terrible." Or tired. Or overwhelmed. Or lost. Or all of these emotions and more.

Understanding the Themes:

Let's begin by dissecting why this scenario is common and why women often mask their emotional struggles following Breast Cancer. One recurring theme is the innate ability of women, in particular, to conceal their emotional distress. Women are adept at maintaining a facade of well-being, even convincing themselves that everything is fine. I mean let's face it, women are genetically geared to be resilient. We have a strong tendency to care for everyone else around us, particularly our children, and place ourselves last. It is uncommon for women to look after themselves as well as they look after others.

The typical response to inquiries about a woman's well-being is a stoic, "I'm fine," even when they may be far from it. However, it often takes considerable time for women to acknowledge how much their mental health has been impacted following a diagnosis of Breast Cancer.

So, if you're reading this chapter, I encourage you to pause for a moment and honestly assess your mental well-being throughout your breast cancer journey. Check-in with yourself regularly throughout your treatment and following.

Some might think, "Well, this doesn't apply to me. My mental health is just fine." And that is perfectly valid. However, the prevalence of this theme among breast cancer patients has prompted me to address it. Particularly considering many women will put on a very brave front for friends, family and colleagues. But even the strongest of women can be affected by the brutality that is Breast Cancer. And there is no shame in admitting it. In actual fact, for those women who consider themselves strong, capable and independent, let me offer my most valuable piece of advice (particularly considering I too consider myself a strong, capable and independent woman)....accept help from others, and know that it is ok to feel fragile, sad, terrified, and weak at times due to your Breast Cancer. Even strong women need help.

The medical focus is often on the physical aspects of breast cancer treatment, such as surgery, chemotherapy, or radiation therapy. Mental health sometimes takes a backseat. This should absolutely not be the case in this day and age, but unfortunately, I still come across way too many women who have never been offered referral to a Psychologist or Counsellor following their Breast Cancer diagnosis. In many cases, there isn't a standardized referral pathway to mental health professionals for every breast cancer patient. While there's great emphasis on addressing physical aspects, we must equally prioritize mental and emotional health during this journey.

The Caregiver Nature of Women:

One factor contributing to this "I'm fine" facade is that women are natural caregivers. They excel at caring for others—children, grandchildren, ageing parents, pets, homes, husbands, and jobs—yet often neglect self-care.

There's a tendency to resist accepting help from others, driven by a sense of independence and appearing capable. It could also be driven by the fact that you've never had anyone to help. Plenty of single mothers, women who are single and widowers are diagnosed with Breast Cancer. Therefore, the first and most crucial advice is to allow others to lend a hand when you need it. This is a recurring theme throughout this chapter because it's essential. It can be a strange thing for a woman to put herself before others, particularly family. Women often tell me they feel selfish when focusing on their own well-being. But to successfully navigate the journey that is Breast Cancer, this action is often necessary.

The Perspective of Others:

It's a journey filled with unknowns and foreign experiences for those who haven't lived it. Understanding this perspective can help ease any frustration you might feel when others offer well-intentioned but misguided comments.

However, if repetitive attempts of offers to help from well-meaning friends or colleagues are becoming a negative force in your journey, it may be best to keep a healthy distance from these types of people. At least until you have regained some mental and physical strength.

It's Okay to Say, "I'm Not Okay"

While many breast cancer patients put on a brave face, expressing when you're not okay is equally important, at least to certain people you trust. You don't have to announce it to the world, but select individuals, including your medical team, should be aware of your emotional struggles. Sometimes, these medical professionals can trigger referrals to mental health specialists, such as counsellors or psychologists, and I will state again that this should be a standard pathway for breast cancer patients. It should be up to the woman diagnosed with Breast Cancer to decline the referral to a mental health professional, not an assumption made by a Medical Professional that the patient may not want or need support for their mental health.

The Road to Empowerment:

In conclusion, this chapter highlights three key issues: the universal tendency for women to hide their emotional struggles despite sometimes dire circumstances, the gap in understanding from people around you who haven't experienced breast cancer, and the lack of a standard pathway for mental health support in breast cancer care. To address these issues, I recommend three strategies:

1. **Seek Out Trusted Allies:** Identify individuals, whether they are family, friends, or members of your medical team, with whom you can openly discuss your mental health. Venting and sharing your emotional journey with these trusted allies can provide significant relief.

2. **Engage in Specialized Exercise:** Consult an exercise specialist experienced in working with breast cancer patients. Physical activity can be a powerful tool in reducing stress, boosting energy levels and triggering endorphin release, promoting a sense of well-being. Exercise specialists can tailor programs to your unique needs.

3. **Mental Health Support:** If your mental health significantly impacts your daily life, don't hesitate to seek help from a mental health professional, such as a counsellor or psychologist. Ideally, choose a professional with experience treating breast cancer patients to ensure specialized care. Alternatively, seek out a local Breast Cancer Support Group and if there isn't an established group in your area, consider online support groups.

Your well-being, both physical and emotional, matters. **By embracing these strategies and acknowledging your emotional needs, you can take a proactive step toward improving your mental health during and after your breast cancer journey.**

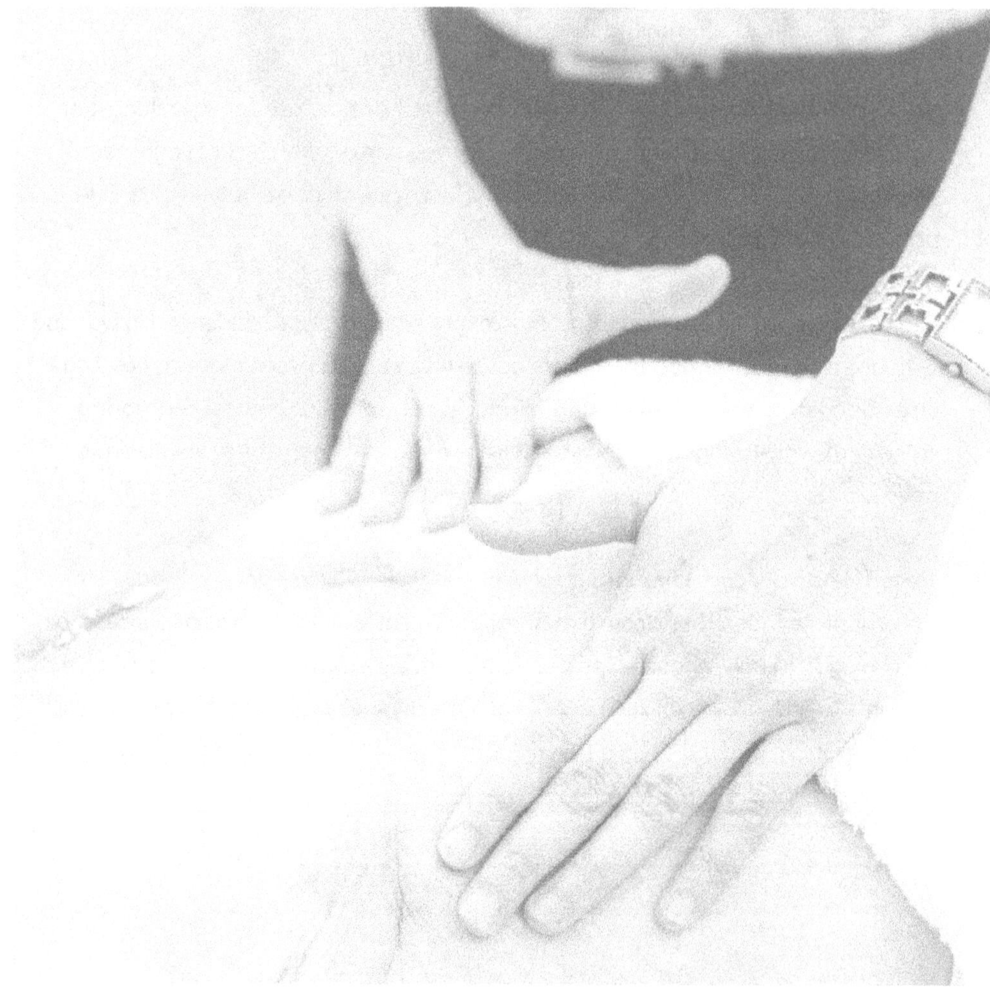

www.BreastCancerRevolution.co

6.2 Overcoming Mental Challenges After Breast Cancer

The last section of this chapter explores a crucial aspect of life after breast cancer-breaking free from the mental challenges that often linger. While I'm not a psychologist or counsellor, I am a physiotherapist who has spent the last decade specializing in caring for breast cancer patients. In that time, I've assisted around 40 breast cancer patients every week, allowing me to identify common themes that arise post-treatment. One such theme is the mental struggle that often follows the completion of active treatment.

After enduring the rigours of breast cancer treatment, it's perfectly understandable to find yourself in a tough mental space. A cancer diagnosis is a significant life event that provides an opportunity for introspection. It forces you to reassess your life and its priorities. While the term "new normal" is often used, I am quick to say I am not the biggest fan of this phrase. Whilst there are certain facts that may be defined as "the new normal", such as being flat-chested after a double mastectomy if you are not undergoing reconstruction, symptoms such as poor exercise tolerance, poor sleep quality or persistent fatigue should not be considered the "new normal" as there are many options for these treatment side effects.

Women are capable of phenomenal things after Breast Cancer, and although some things may have changed forever, there are many examples of lingering symptoms that have not yet had enough recovery time or the appropriate treatment applied, and should not be considered your "new normal".

I encourage you to view Breast Cancer as an opportunity to create version 2.0 of yourself.

Consider what you would like to change in your life following your diagnosis that might bring more energy, joy and purpose. Embrace the chance to become a more resilient and empowered individual. I'd like to share five essential strategies to help you improve your mental well-being after breast cancer:

1. **Exercise for Mental Health:** Exercise is a powerful tool for enhancing mental health. It triggers the release of endorphins, helping alleviate depression and boosting overall mood. Integrating exercise into your routine can significantly improve your mental well-being, such as a daily walk, joining a fitness group, hitting the gym, or practising yoga. I particularly recommend resistance training for its multitude of benefits following Breast Cancer treatment.

2. **Prioritize Quality Sleep:** Quality sleep is vital for mental health. Breast cancer survivors often face sleep disturbances, which treatments like hormone blockers can exacerbate. Addressing these issues, whether through exercise, medication adjustments or implementing good sleep hygiene practices can make a significant difference.

3. **Seek Mental Health Support:** Don't hesitate to seek support when your mental health is suffering. Joining breast cancer support groups or engaging with counsellors or psychologists can provide invaluable guidance. It's essential to break the stigma surrounding mental health and prioritize your well-being.

4. **Change Your Routine:**

5. **Address Lingering Symptoms:** Finally, addressing lingering symptoms is crucial. Ignoring ongoing pain, mobility issues or cognitive challenges can exacerbate your mental rut. Work with your healthcare team to find solutions, whether through physical therapy, occupational therapy, or other specialized care.

EPILOGUE

In this first volume of Breast Cancer Revolution, I have endeavoured to provide valuable insights and guidance on the multifaceted journey of breast cancer recovery. We've explored the critical role of physiotherapy in your healing process, emphasizing the importance of a single physio appointment as an essential step. We've discussed physical recovery after surgery, helping you embrace freedom through a range of movement exercises.

Understanding lymphoedema and its prevention has been a significant focus, with discussions on recognizing its signs, assessing your risk, and following current guidelines. We've harnessed the empowering benefits of exercise and lymphatic drainage, providing you with tools to kickstart your fitness journey and manage swelling.

Perhaps most importantly, we've addressed breast cancer survivors' often-overlooked mental challenges. From coping with the dissonance between appearance and inner feelings to breaking free from the mental rut, we've discussed strategies to restore your inner radiance and resilience.

Throughout these chapters, I have aimed to inspire and support you on your path to recovery. Your strength and courage are evident in every step you take; this volume is a tribute to your indomitable spirit. Remember, this is just the beginning of your journey toward renewed health and inner radiance, and I am honoured to be a part of it.

American Society of Clinical Oncology, Cancer.Net (2023) Breast Cancer Statistics. https://www.cancer.net/cancer-types/breast-cancer/statistics

Boehnke Michaud L. & Goodin S. (2006) Cancer-treatment-induced bone loss, part 1. American Journal of Health-System Pharmacy 63:419-430

Cormie P., Atkinson, M., Bucci L., Cust A., Eakin E., Hayes S., McCarthy S., Murnane A., Patchell S. & Adams D. (2018) Clinical Oncology Society of Australia Position Statement on exercise in cancer care. Medical Journal of Australia 209: 184-187

Downs T.L., Whiteside E.J., Foot G., Mills D.E., Bliss E.S. (2023) Differences in total cognition and cerebrovascular function in female breast cancer survivors and cancer-free women. The Breast 69:358-365

Heydon-White H., Suami H., Boyages J., Koelmeyer L., Peebles K. (2020) Assessing breast lymphoedema following breast cancer treatment using indocyanine green lymphography. Breast Cancer Research and Treatment 181: 635-644

Koelmeyer L.A., Thompson B.M., Mackie H., Blackwell R., Heydon-White A., Moloney E., Gaitatzis K., Boyages J., Suami H. (2020) Personalizing Conservative Lymphedema Management Using Indocyanine Green-Guided Manual Lymphatic Drainage. Lymphatic Research and Biology 00: 1-10

Schmitz K.H., Troxel A.B., Cheville A., Grant L.L., Bryan C.J., Gross C.R., Lytle L.A., & Ahmed R.L. (2009) Physical Activity and Lymphedema (the PAL trial): Assessing the safety of progressive strength training in breast cancer survivors. Contemporary Clinical Trials 30:233-245